The First Year

# OUT

# The First Year OUT

## Mental Patients after Hospitalization

William W. Michaux
Martin M. Katz
Albert A. Kurland
Kathleen H. Gansereit

The Johns Hopkins Press, Baltimore

Standard Book Number 8018-1057-4



Manufactured in the United States of America

Library of Congress Catalog Card Number 74-78346

# Foreword

New developments in social psychiatry and psychopharmacology have greatly altered the composition of state hospital patient populations and the life experience of the severely mentally ill. As emphasis in treatment of patients shifts to the community, we see changes in the diagnostic, demographic, and symptomatic characteristics of patients who enter the state hospitals. This contributes to radical changes in the character of the institution itself and modifies the state hospital's place in the overall treatment picture. The role of the state hospital is slowly but surely being redefined. Like many "total treatments" before it, it is evolving into something quite different, unfortunately, before we have had time to evaluate its therapeutic impact as a self-contained program. Increases in discharge rates have, in many instances, become tragically balanced by proportionate increases in readmission rates. It is this paradox—and our lack of knowledge concerning the durability of in-hospital treatments—that have served to stimulate numerous investigations concerning the posthospital experiences of the mentally ill.

Research represents a quest for those variables that might predict both the patient's tenure in the community and the level of his personal and social adjustment. The results, unfortunately, are sometimes ambiguous, often contradictory, and frequently fragmented. Most often, these deficiencies can be traced to limitations in study design, to sheer practical difficulties of conducting long-term research in the community, and to inadequacies of our methods of measurement. The reasons for these deficiencies and for the dearth of follow-up studies in general are understandable. Longitudinal studies of posthospital adjustment and effects of treatment do not permit the kind of control over the patients' lives and treatment experiences that can be provided within the hospital. In contrast to the laboratory-like setting of the hospital, a community setting introduces many different and complicated logistic and practical problems in measurement, and in reaching the patients at predetermined intervals following their discharge.

Even where it is possible to overcome all the practical problems of contact with patients, such as gaining the cooperation of key informants or maintaining close and systematic communication with them over a lengthy period of time, there still remains the critical problem of how and what to measure. Which patient characteristics and which situational characteristics are worthy of measurement? How do we define clinical, personal, and social adjustment? What variables provide the kind of information that is essential for making progress in understanding the process of mental disorder and its various manifestations over time? What historical, environmental, and personal variables alter the course of the disorder in the direction of either survival in the community or rehospitalization? These questions involve complicated methodologic issues and require establishment of comprehensive measures of "adjustment" which encompass broad definitions of mental disorder and mental health. Further, the patient's progress cannot be measured by a simple indication of how he looks one year after discharge: this requires an intensity of measurement hitherto untried.

Most attempts, then, to understand the tenure and adjustment of former inpatients have resembled rather an archeological probe through the layers of human suffering and social dysfunction than a systematic, concurrent, and prospective scrutiny of an individual's life after hospitalization. This volume presents an alternative to such post-hoc investigations, both in methodology and focus of inquiry.

Month by month, through the first year out, the reader is invited to serve as a non-participant observer, a witness to the course of adjustment of 139 patients. Who are these patients, what does their course of adjustment look like? Who gets treated, who does not? Who does well, who does poorly? Who survives, who fails? These questions are approached in the context of time; the answers are neither predictable nor always pleasant.

In a unique manner, early posthospital experiences are used to predict adjustment and rehospitalization one year later. Aspects of symptomatology and the patients' and relatives' expectations and their satisfaction are assessed one month following discharge and related to subsequent adjustment at one year. The level and quality of the patients' early—and poor—social behavior is seen as a catalyst interacting with an environment that ultimately rejects and hospitalizes the patient. In view of these findings, previous claims that discount the relationship between role performance, social behavior, and rehospitalization must now be reexamined, if not abandoned.

Within the fabric of predictions about adjustment, pertinent features of past history, life situation variables, and current environmental stressors are carefully interwoven. The patterns which emerge are distinct; they differ depending upon whether one wishes to explain adjustment or rehospitalization.

Here is an anthology to be used repeatedly by those who wish to treat, prevent, or explore the residuals of disorder and the effects of hospitalization among the mentally ill.

BERTRAM S. BROWN, M.D.
*Deputy Director*
*National Institute of Mental Health*

# Preface

The research here reported was conducted at Spring Grove State Hospital near Baltimore, Maryland. The project was supported by PHS Research Grant No. MH 05529 from the National Institute of Mental Health, Public Health Service. Friends of Psychiatric Research, Inc., managed the grant and provided substantial help in project administration. The authors' roles were as follows: Dr. William W. Michaux, Project Director; Dr. Martin M. Katz, National Institute of Mental Health Staff Consultant; Dr. Albert A. Kurland, Principal Investigator; and Kathleen H. Gansereit, Research Associate. The project's Co-principal Investigator was Dr. Thomas E. Hanlon.

We acknowledge with gratitude the cooperation of Dr. Bruno Radauskas, Superintendent of Spring Grove State Hospital, and Dr. Aris M. Simopoulos, former Clinical Director. Smith Kline and French Laboratories kindly supplied copies of their pamphlet, *A New Chapter*, for distribution to patients.

The tasks which we set for ourselves in designing the study entailed some rather formidable and unusual difficulties, particularly in regard to collecting and processing longitudinal data on volunteer subjects living in widely scattered Maryland homes. Now that the job is done and we look back on its ardors and vicissitudes, we are convinced that our schemes would have quietly come to naught, had it not been for exceptionally high-caliber collaboration. To recognize the diverse contributions of those who furthered this work is therefore more than a formality; it is a counting of blessings and a fond recollection.

We think first of Anita Gilbert, whose untimely death cut short the bounty of her social-work skills. Among other staff members, the Examiners all contributed decisively: Richard D. Cameron, Dr. David G. Crough, Henry L. Hammond, and Dr. Oliver L. McCabe. In bringing the project to a close, Kristan A. Rodger as Research Associate was our prime mover in computer liaison and manuscript work. Doretha M. Brown, Secretary, handled most other office work including initial and specially scheduled evaluation appointments.

From time to time, in addition to these durable staff members, several other employees of Spring Grove State Hospital's Research Department helped temporarily but indispensably with data collection, compilation, and analysis. They were George F. Kopits, Ruth L. Jones, Marilyn K. Rosenstein, Sondra R. Tepper, and Leola A. Tracey.

Many of our subjects were attending the Outpatient Clinic at the hospital. Dr. Gertrude J. Fleischmann and her clinic staff are especially to be thanked for enabling us frequently to conduct our research evaluation sessions in conjunction with treatment appointments. Similar arrangements at other clinics were facilitated by Helen Tighe. At Spring Grove State Hospital, Lee Wright and her co-workers were most obliging in making available medical records, and Genevieve Wagoner was constantly helpful with library service.

Countless professional judgments and decisions had to be made in planning and executing the project—at times with scant if any precedent. In this area we owe substantial credit to senior colleagues—in particular to Dr. Jonathan O. Cole, Dr. Gertrude J. Fleischmann, Gerard E. Hogarty, Hubertine Marshall, Dr. Charles Savage, and Dr. Mary H. Michaux who was also a steadfast editorial helpmeet.

The Maryland Psychiatric Case Register contained data which proved most useful in dealing with the problems of sampling bias.

Dr. Kurt Gorwitz and Mr. William Phillips generously provided us the necessary information on the patients in question.

In processing our data we were ably assisted by James A. Forbes, Henri A. Lowery, Dr. John W. Shaffer, and Dr. Antanas Suziedelis. Their special skills and their personal interest in the work did much to maximize the yield of findings here conveyed.

WILLIAM W. MICHAUX, PH.D.

Baltimore, Maryland

# Contents*

* An asterisk designates each section or subsection dealing mainly with methodology, for the benefit of readers interested in this aspect of the study but of less interest to readers who concentrate on its clinical and social aspects.

Chapter I

# Design and Procedure

In recent years many researchers have studied the psychiatric patient's adjustment and social functioning during the critical months following hospitalization. Yet the posthospital year as a continuous, changing experience remains incompletely charted. The deficit has been due in large part to formidable practical difficulties of longitudinal data collection and a scarcity of suitable assessment techniques. Confronting such limitations, investigators have tended to focus on a few decisive occasions such as discharge, rehospitalization, and discharge anniversaries. Otherwise, scant attention has been paid to changes in the patient during the follow-up period. Moreover, many posthospital evaluations have been retrospective and hence of questionable usefulness for prediction within their adopted time spans.

From one or another standpoint the present study resembles earlier ones, notably those by Angrist, Dinitz, Lefton, and Pasamanick (1961); Dinitz, Angrist, Lefton, and Pasamanick (1961); Freeman and Simmons (1963); Gorwitz, Bahn, Klee, and Solomon (1966); Marks, Stauffacher, and Lyle (1963); and Orlinsky and D'Elia (1964). It is a systematic field study emphasizing psychosocial variables; it does not purport to evaluate the effects of inpatient treatment per se; tests and interviews are used to assess patients; and the general objective is to increase clinical knowledge concerning posthospital adjustment and rehospitalization.

## PURPOSES AND INNOVATIONS

In other respects our study is unique in its genre. It was conceived as an intensive longitudinal investigation of the *course* of in-community clinical and social adjustment manifested by typical ex-patients of a state mental hospital. It aims toward defining more precisely the preconditions and hallmarks of successful *vs.* unsuccessful adjustment, and toward developing guidelines and hypotheses for subsequent investigation with tighter controls. While no direct effort is made to test the effects of the aftercare treatment which many of the patients received, such treatment is closely surveyed in context. Prevention of (further) hospitalization is an issue to which our findings are premeditatedly relevant.

Given this outlook, the investigation took shape methodologically as a deliberate venture in constructive innovation. Its success could not be guaranteed in advance; but as it turned out, the adequacy of collected data exceeded conservative forecasts. Thus, the study constitutes not merely a body of findings but also a trial demonstration of novel methods applicable to controlled evaluation of either inpatient or outpatient treatment. Too often evaluations of inpatient treatment effects rely on assessments made while the patient is still hospitalized and stop short of the ultimately decisive outcome, adjustment upon return to the community. Similarly, research in outpatient treatment has tended to underemphasize home and community adjustment as criteria; it is easier, though not necessarily more important or conclusive, to assess the patient with standard general-purpose tests of personality, or with measurements bounded by the clinic, its intramural professional observers, and the patient's visits. In vitro measurements are heuristically essential; in the area here under study, however, we are proportionately oversupplied with the likes of them and must begin to round out the incomplete links of knowledge in vivo.

The methodological novelty stemming from this rationale is threefold: (1) characteristics of the sample, (2) longitudinal coverage, (3) measurement techniques. What is unique to the study is its strategic combination of the following features within a single protocol, not that the features are themselves all unprecedented.

*1. Characteristics of the Sample.* Subject to several selection criteria, a determined effort was made to obtain a random, representative sample of ex-patients of a single state mental hospital, limited diagnostically to nonorganic illnesses. Supplementally, a special study was conducted to assay the nature and extent of sampling bias. Furthermore, our volunteer subjects began as noninstitutionalized individuals who were simply living at large in communities near the hospital; though many were in aftercare treatment, selection was without regard to their attendance at outpatient treatment centers. (Details of sampling and other procedures are set forth later in this chapter.)

*2. Longitudinal Coverage.* To achieve fine-grained, chronologically continuous coverage of all in-community time during the posthospital year, our design stipulated 12 monthly evaluations with repeated use of the same tests and interview forms. Each of these evaluations encompassed the entire preceding month.

*3. Measurement Techniques.* The multidimensional evaluations of clinical and social adjustment were reasonably comprehensive. They employed previously validated questionnaires specifically designed for assessing psychiatric patients in the community. Central to their conception was the use of a lay informant, usually a close relative of the subject, as observer and reporter of clinically meaningful aspects of patient behavior, complementing the self-report obtained directly from the patient. In addition, monthly interviews with both parties provided basic information on the patient's ongoing life situation not only at home but also (when applicable) at work and in treatment. Finally, the same interviews also undertook to measure recent and current environmental stress.

Clearly, then, our investigative design was heterodox, although many of its features mimicked well-established methods. And the hazards which it posed for data collection reappeared as special issues in interpretation of the results. For these reasons we shall, throughout the report, have more to say and exhibit pertaining to methodology and logistics than is usually the case. Of particular concern are logistical problems encountered in the effort to cover all possible in-community time, as well as organizational problems in handling obtained data despite gaps due both to rehospitalization and to sporadic noncompletion of scheduled evaluations.

## SPRING GROVE STATE HOSPITAL

Spring Grove State Hospital, where all of our ex-patients had previously been admitted, is a large, long-established, moderately progressive public mental institution. It is located in Catonsville, Maryland, just southwest of the Baltimore city line. It routinely admits all kinds of adult psychiatric patients except mental defectives and convicted criminals. Selected child cases comprise a very small segment of its population. Racial desegregation of admissions had barely begun when we initiated data collection in February 1963; at that time the hospital had very few Negro inpatients.

Spring Grove is one of four major state mental hospitals serving Maryland, each with its own catchment areas. To Spring Grove are admitted all patients from Baltimore County (which adjoins but does not overlap Baltimore City), Cecil County, Harford County, and Prince George's County. Also eligible for admission are those Baltimore City patients residing in postal zones 7, 23, 26, 27, 28, 29, 30, and 36.[1] During fiscal year 1964 (July, 1963 through June, 1964), when our project was in midstream, the hospital's average daily patient population was 2,438. In the same year, a total of 2,606 patients were admitted and 2,362 were discharged. The hospital's diversified treatment program emphasizes drug therapy and milieu therapy, and includes aftercare, social service, occupational therapy, vocational rehabilitation, individual and group psychotherapy, and recreation supervised by volunteer workers.

Recent state-wide trends for public psychiatric hospital treatment in Maryland resemble those of the nation in some respects; at the same time there are noteworthy differences. The Maryland Department of Mental Hygiene (1966) observed that, for the six years 1958-1964:

[1] A few of the patients in our study may have resided elsewhere in Maryland, inasmuch as Spring Grove's catchment areas have varied from time to time. At the present writing, they are not exactly the same as designated here.

> Maryland's admission and net release rates are considerably higher and are increasing at a faster rate than in the rest of the country. In Maryland, also, the average patient population rate decreased 25 per cent during the six year period (from 320.5 to 239.6 per 100,000 total state population while the decline in the rest of the United States was only 18 per cent (from 308.7 to 262.7). These data would indicate that Maryland hospitals treat and return to the community a proportionally greater number of patients. . . . Although Maryland's per patient expenditure continued to exceed the national average, its relative rank declined slightly since 1958. That is, the number of states with a higher average expenditure is increasing.

The average length of a single hospitalization in Maryland has decreased. More hospital beds have come to be occupied by acutely ill patients, and fewer by the chronically ill who formerly predominated. Geographically, admission rates are inordinately high for the deteriorated "inner city" area of Baltimore, with its formidable economic, social, and public health problems typical of American urban centers. Gorwitz (1966) notes that "more than 35,000, or one per cent, of Maryland's residents receive treatment in a psychiatric facility [including outpatient clinics] at some time during a one-year period. This rate has increased in recent years."

Our project staff offices were located in the hospital's main admission building. Clinical records on patients, which we consulted for our data, were also kept in this building. The project workers were members of a large interdisciplinary Research Department founded in 1953 and housed in various buildings mostly on the hospital grounds (Kurland, 1954; Kurland, 1962). All personnel who worked directly on the project were full-time employees and had no other duties. The study was planned in 1962; its formal operating period covered five years beginning in January 1963.

## *SAMPLING PROCEDURE

A sample of potential subjects was drawn from the official Spring Grove records of all currently released patients. Adults of both sexes were accepted, regardless of their participation or nonparticipation in any form of aftercare treatment. The only requirement as to prior inpatient status was that the subject must have spent at least one night at Spring Grove, with or without treatment of any kind. There was no restriction on type of admission or on number, length, or place of earlier hospitalizations. Our sampling for the study proper, excluding trial-run cases, began with patients who left the hospital in February, 1963. The last patients selected left in July, 1964 and finished their study year in July, 1965.

The following seven criteria governed our selection of newly released patients:

*1. Age.* To be eligible for the study, a patient must have been at least 18 when he or she left the hospital. There was no upper age limit. Thus the full range of adulthood was sampled.

*2. Race.* Negroes were excluded. When the study began, the hospital had, as noted, not achieved complete desegregation. The patient population was predominantly white.

*3. Diagnosis.* The patient's final primary hospital diagnosis, and also any secondary diagnosis on record, must have been one of the "disorders of psychogenic origin" as classified in the APA diagnostic manual (American Psychiatric Association, 1952). However, two diagnoses in this group, alcoholism and drug addiction, were excluded because of the addict's distinctive psychosocial problems which require equally distinctive methods for evaluation. With these two exceptions, our sample covered potentially the full range of the functional psychiatric disorders: psychoses, psychophysiologic disorders, neuroses, personality disorders, and transient situational personality disorders. Mental deficiency was entirely excluded, as were brain disorders both acute and chronic.

*4. Type of Hospital Release.* This sampling criterion was important as a control on the patient's posthospital social situation. The only two acceptable types of release, and their conditions as defined administratively by the hospital, were (a) discharge with doctor's consent—a closing of the case with no continuation of hospital responsibility; and (b) convalescent leave—a provisional discharge, usually for one year, allowing readmission with very little paper work, and convertible at expiration either to outright discharge or to extended convalescent leave. By excluding all other types of release we ensured that every patient to be studied was leaving the hospital with medical sanction, was considered to have a reasonable chance of remaining out for at least a year, and was free to resume ordinary home and community living without major clinical or legal restrictions. These requirements disqualified any patient who, for example, had been released from the hospital to a foster home, to court custody, on temporary home visit (trial visit), or against medical advice.

*5. Location of Residence.* The patient's posthospital residence had to be in Maryland and not more than 60 miles from the hospital. The in-state requirement was adopted to avoid jurisdictional complications. The 60-mile limit was the maximum distance that participants or staff could reasonably be expected to travel for monthly evaluations. We estimate that, despite these territorial restrictions, we sampled from at least 96 per cent of the Spring Grove ex-patient population, as defined by contemporaneous statistics (U.S. Department of Health, Education, and Welfare, and Maryland State Department of Mental Hygiene, 1964, Vol. 1, p. 19; Vol. 2, p. 13). According to the state figures, the majority of our few geographically excluded patients were probably out-of-state residents. Most of the in-state territory which exceeded our 60-mile limit was served by state hospitals other than Spring Grove.

*6. Time Out of Hospital.* Following his last pre-study hospitalization, the patient must have remained unrehospitalized for at least the first 20 consecutive days. This requirement was necessitated by several interlocking practical considerations. While one could argue that ideally it should not have been observed as a criterion of eligibility for study, it actually eliminated only three patients who would otherwise have been eligible. It is true that this particular subclass of patients is often considered to be highly vulnerable and hence to merit special study. From another viewpoint, however, one can hold that, in terms of the discharge decision, these patients were "false starts"—individuals who were clinically misjudged as to their readiness for community living. At any rate, the definition of our sample as regards those patients who became rehospitalized during the posthospital study year must contain the qualifying clause implied by our 20-days-out requirement.

One practical consideration which determined the 20-day criterion was based on project-design requirements. We had stipulated that, while we would have to tolerate some incompleteness of data due to inevitable missed evaluations, every patient to be studied must complete the first-month evaluation for use as baseline data. Thus, we knew in advance that a patient could become rehospitalized even before we had finished our screening and recruiting.

A second reality consideration interacted with this limitation. It proved impossible, albeit desirable, to screen patients for the study before they had actually left the hospital. In the local clinical practice of discharging patients from any of numerous buildings, the length of time between decision and action was in many instances much too short to permit effective co-ordination of research machinery with the normal daily flow of clinical work. Furthermore, we learned in our pre-study trial run that a 20-day post-discharge waiting period was often necessary to assure that the clinical information essential to us had been recorded in the patient's file.

7. *Handicap.* The patient and also the informant had to be free of any serious physical or language handicap which might hinder testing or interviewing. If a patient was testable despite being handicapped, a second requirement was that his disability should be judged not to preclude reasonably adequate social functioning; otherwise he would have been unfairly disadvantaged in the evaluations. Blindness, for example, was considered a prohibitive physical handicap in this respect. One or two persons of foreign extraction, with little or no command of spoken English, were linguistically disqualified because they would have been unable to communicate adequately with the examiner.

For each patient who became identified as a candidate for the study, a willing and suitable informant also had to be recruited. We observed the same minimum age limit of 18 for informants as for patients. In seeking the most suitable informant our general order of preference was (1) the patient's spouse, (2) a parent, (3) a sibling, (4) a son or daughter, (5) any other relative, and (6) a close friend or other non-relative. Not acceptable as informants were clinicians or others whose prime relationship with the patient was professional rather than personal.

Another aspect of the patient-informant relationship which required careful attention was the adequacy of contact between the two parties. The optimum informant in this respect was the one who lived under the same roof with the patient and kept in daily personal touch with him. Almost all of our informants saw the patients at least daily. Our minimum standard for patient-informant interaction, to ensure adequate observation of the patient, was several contacts per month, involving something more than casual conversation.

Figure I-1 illustrates the flow of patients from hospital release, through various classifications, to the end of the follow-up year. Lettered boxes are patient classifications; numbered steps are research operations. For clarity, the sketch is simplified; it does not show, for example, that a relapser patient could become also a reneger *after* re-entering and leaving the hospital.[2]

In order to regulate the rate of accession of eligible patients and obtain a representative sample of manageable size, we randomly selected candidates from the total flow of eligibles. We adopted two interlocking methods of randomization: skipping patients by drawing lots, and skipping release dates on the basis of expediency.

For a given release date which was *not* to be skipped, our starting point for sampling (Figure I-1, step 1) was the hospital's daily list of all patients who had left. We usually screened these lists in units of two consecutive days for convenience and economy. Every patient listed was classified as eligible or ineligible for the study by reference to hospital records, our seven sampling criteria, and other sources of information as needed. (Occasionally, a patient's ineligi-

[2]The standard term "test," which appears in the figure and throughout the report, is used for brevity to denote a single complete monthly evaluation undergone by patient and informant. Each party completed a questionnaire and was interviewed by the examiner. Details of the evaluation procedure are given below in this chapter.

One other repeated word usage calls for clarification at this point. When referring to a patient in the abstract, we write "he" as obliged by custom. Nevertheless, as will be seen, females outnumbered males in the study sample.

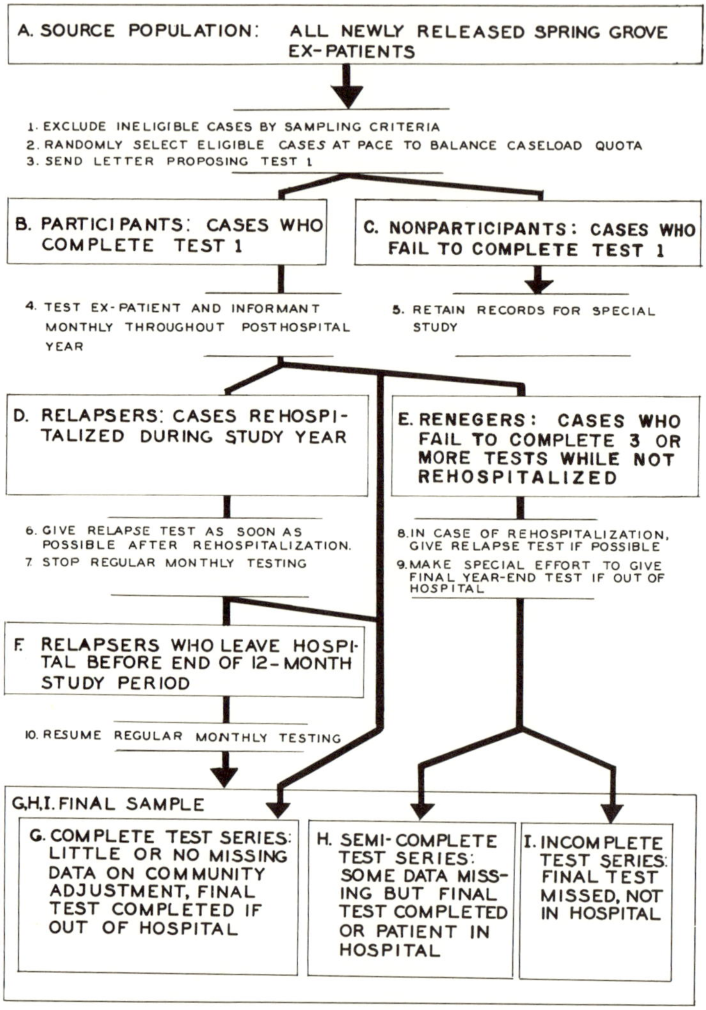


**Figure I-1. Design and procedure of the study.**

bility would not become evident until a later stage of processing, whereupon he was then removed from the study.)

Having compiled the periodic list of eligible patients, we next eliminated excess cases, when necessary, by drawing lots (Figure I-1, step 2). Excess cases were any number of patients above a current predetermined quota which available staff could begin evaluating on schedule. We eliminated a total of 35 eligible patients in this manner, as against 218 potential subjects selected. Thus, 84 per cent of all individuals identified as eligible acceded to the study's starting roster. An additional 36 patients who had left the hospital could not be classified as to eligibility because of misplaced or lost records or because some items of information, e.g., final diagnosis, were not obtainable in time to schedule and conduct the first posthospital evaluation. (These and all other counts do not include 15 trial-run subjects who were processed in a preparatory phase in order to refine and standardize our procedures. Three of the trial-run subjects completed the same 12-month evaluation series as most of those evaluated in the main sample.)

Daily rosters of patients released from the hospital were screened on 208 days (39.0 per cent) out of the total of 533 days which elapsed from the beginning of sampling in February, 1963 to termination in July, 1964. We suspended daily screening whenever the current research caseload was at a maximum. There was no bias as to particular days of the week skipped. The major suspension of screening was for 151 consecutive days between September, 1963 and February, 1964; during the latter month the earliest cases finished their study year, began to be closed, and could be replaced with newly recruited subjects. Thus, of necessity, sampling was conducted in two waves separated by a five-month waiting period.

What proportion of the parent population did our sample constitute? Was the representation proportionately balanced as between the first and second waves? We selected our 218 candidates at an average rate of 1.0 per day—a pace far slower than that of the total exodus from the hospital. We can answer the two questions very approximately by using Spring Grove statistics released monthly through the Maryland Psychiatric Case Register (Gorwitz, Bahn, Chandler, and Martin, 1963). The Case Register statistics overestimate the size of our true parent population of Spring Grove ex-patients, for the reason that they comprise *all* patients leaving Spring Grove on convalescent leave or discharge during each month of our active sampling; that is, adjustments were not possible for any of our screening criteria except type of release. Of a total of 2,754 patients leaving Spring Grove during these months, our 218 candidates comprised 7.9 per cent; the percentage for the true parent population would of course be higher, perhaps twice as high. Considering the first and second wave time periods separately, we find identical percentages of 7.9 for our two waves as against the respective total exodus rates. The Case Register release count was 1,487 for the first wave period (54.0 per cent of the total 2,754); for the second wave period the total count was 1,267 (46.0 per cent).

## *OBTAINING PARTICIPATION: TEST 1

The study design called for each patient and informant to report monthly on the patient's community adjustment and life situation throughout the first posthospital year. Time spent in a mental hospital via readmission was counted in the posthospital year, but was not covered by the reports, since adjustment in the community was the focus of study. If a rehospitalized patient returned home before his year ended, we resumed monthly testing to complete his interrupted 12-month follow-up. Thus, except when scheduled tests were missed, all of the patient's time in the community throughout his first posthospital year was evaluated longitudinally by monthly retrospective reports.

Our initial request to the patient dealt only with the Month-1 test. Later tests were proposed only after Test 1 had been completed; this approach was designed to minimize initial resistance and refusal. To solicit participation in the first test, we sent the patient a form letter several days before his 30th posthospital day (Figure I-1, step 3; see also Appendix A). It indicated a tentative appointment time and place and explained what was involved, including the need for an accompanying informant. An optional $5.00 reimbursement was offered to cover travel to our office or related expenses. Although we freely used home visits for the later tests, we exerted moderate pressure for an office appointment for Test 1. By having both the patient and the informant visit the research office at this time, we could, we felt, more ably solicit their participation in the additional 11 months of follow-up. Time was of the essence in the entire process of screening, selecting, and recruiting subjects, since Test 1 was required for everyone as a baseline measure and since it had to be completed between the patient's 20th and 40th posthospital days inclusive—preferably on his 30th day.

A few days before our proposed date for Test 1, the project secretary routinely telephoned the patient, hopefully to confirm the appointment for him and his informant. From this point onward the recruiting procedure and outcome depended on the other party's response. As was expected, responses ranged from concurrence plus completion of Test 1, through rescheduling the appointment and then keeping or missing it, to outright refusal even when as a last resort we offered to have our examiner visit the home for Test 1 (Figure I-1, boxes B and C). In some of the nonparticipant cases no response whatever was elicited from the patient—typically when he had no telephone or had moved and left no forwarding address. Whatever the complications, we made every reasonable effort to contact and persuade each individual. At times it became necessary to talk with a potential informant at this stage, either to deal with the patient's reluctance or to help him in arranging a second party's participation.

## *OBTAINING PARTICIPATION: TESTS 2-12

Monthly tests Nos. 2 through 12 were sought only for those cases where both patient and informant completed Test 1. All other cases selected for study were classed as "nonparticipants—no test data"; they were evaluated later in a separate round of data collection (Figure I-1, steps 4 and 5).

Immediately after the completion of Test 1, the project director talked with the patient and informant together and disclosed the longitudinal nature of the study. Whenever the project director was absent, as on all home visits, the examiner handled this phase of recruiting. To document the explanation and to help establish a meaningful working-together relationship for the year-long stretch, we gave the patient at this time a specially prepared mimeographed leaflet titled "The Community Follow-Up Survey" (see Appendix B). In question-and-answer format, the leaflet described the nature and purpose of the study from the patient and informant's standpoint. When handing it to the patient, we suggested that the informant also might wish to read it. Along with this booklet we also gave the patient a copy of *A New Chapter* (Smith Kline & French Laboratories, 1962)—a twelve-page illustrated lay message giving helpful suggestions for recently hospitalized mental patients.

Our proposal at this point was for the patient and informant to continue our identically repeated monthly evaluations for the remainder of the posthospital year. Ideally, all of each patient's time in the community during the year would thus be evaluated in consecutive monthly segments. For those who consented, we made an appointment for the next test upon completion of each current test except the final one, for Month 12.

## *RESEARCH SCHEDULE: MONTHS 2-12

Rehospitalization and, secondarily, participants' unavailability were the two causes of missed tests for Months 2 through 12. Rehospitalization misses were considered legitimate as well as unavoidable in our design, since community adjustment was the subject of study. Unavailability of either patient or informant after Test 1 was the factor which resulted in unjustifiably missed tests in about one-third of our cases. Thus, regardless of whether or not a participant missed any tests, the case when closed was classifiable either as a relapser (rehospitalized during the follow-up year) or nonrelapser.

For relapsers (Figure I-1, box D), a special "relapse test" was required of both patient and informant as soon as possible after readmission to the hospital. Only by this procedure could we close the gap in longitudinal coverage between the last prior "regular test" and readmission—a period generally considered crucial in the course of mental illness. Unlike the regular test, a relapse test could cover as little time as one day or as much as about 29 days. After this evaluation, for as long as the patient remained in the hospital, testing was interrupted. It was resumed if, during his posthospital year as originally determined, he returned home and remained in the community for 20 consecutive days (Figure I-1, steps 6, 7, and 10). (The only exception to this procedure was for a very few elopements; these were considered, for study purposes, to be still hospitalized.) In case of repeated rehospitalization, either before the 20th day out or at any time later in the year, additional relapse testing was done.

An entirely separate procedure was needed whenever tests were missed unjustifiably, i.e., for any reason other than rehospitalization. Once a patient and informant had joined the sample by taking Test 1, either one or both parties might miss any number of tests from none to 11. Actual performances proved almost as diverse as the logical possibilities. Our scheme for handling missed tests was an attempt at sensible compromise between this extreme diversity and the ideal of uniformity which any controlled investigation must at least approximate. We adopted three ground rules, all conservative, to curtail some of the potential asymmetry in the body of obtained data: (1) Whenever any participant had unjustifiably missed three tests, consecutive or otherwise, he was classed as a "reneger"–meaning that further testing was to be attempted only for relapse tests and for Test 12 (Figure I-1: box E, steps 8 and 9). (2) A test missed by either of the two parties was equivalent to one missed by both; the other party's completed test was not to be credited. (3) If the critical relapse test were missed, subsequent monthly tests which were skipped because of continuing hospitalization would be counted as *unjustifiably* missed (instead of legitimately), and the degree of incompleteness for the yearly series would be adjudged on this basis.

Our design placed a premium not only on Test 1, but also on Test 12. By obtaining these two sets of data we would at least be able to study beginning-of-year status and end-of-year status, even in patients who had missed some or all of the intervening tests. We therefore made a special effort to get every participant evaluated at Month 12. For the most part this posed problems only among renegers. The typical extreme in this group was the patient who said he wanted to withdraw from the longitudinal plan, either immediately after taking Test 1 or later. When persuasion failed, and as a last resort at the moment of outspoken withdrawal, we asked if the patient and informant would promise to take only Test 12, when it came due. For all cases, our effort to obtain Test 12 was augmented whenever that test was resisted and was adapted to each individual situation.

Ideally, every test from 2 through 12 would have been administered at 30-day intervals or, to be exact, on each patient's "optimum date," i.e., the same calendar day of each month as the day the patient had left the hospital. To limit variation in appointment dates, we stipulated a minimum and maximum of 20 to 40 days between any two consecutive tests.

Any description of research design and procedure is of necessity schematic and abstract. In being so, it excludes many operational details which may vitally affect the conduct and outcome of the investigation. To give the reader a realistic "feel" for what actually happened in our data collection, we present in Appendix C and, supplementally, Appendix D a complete narrative of the actions involved in following one of our cases throughout her posthospital study year.

## *TESTING ARRANGEMENTS: PLACE, INFORMANT, AND EXAMINER

In a field study, the collection of data must proceed without benefit of many of the built-in controls of the clinical institution or the experimental laboratory. At the same time, scientific orderliness must be preserved in the face of real and pressing demands for procedural resiliency. In the present study, this issue made itself felt not only in terms of formal design as noted above, but also in the tangible details of obtaining the patients' and informants' reports.

One such detail was the question of where to conduct the monthly evaluation sessions. For Test 1, as we have said, our preference was our own offices, but we would visit the home rather than lose the patient. In encouraging participants to come to the office we were favored by being located in the same building with the Spring Grove State Hospital Outpatient Clinic, which provided aftercare to many of our patients. Thus, if a patient had a clinic appointment at the appropriate time, he could, on the same visit, meet our Test-1 request merely by bringing an informant with him and walking down the hall. The same was true for later tests, and an incidental but important advantage was that clinic treatment often followed the same monthly schedule as our follow-up. For all tests after Test 1, however, the option of office, home, or elsewhere was left entirely to the participants. If circumstances made it difficult for patient and informant to appear together, we conducted separate sessions. This was usually the case, for example, for the relapse test: the rehospitalized patient would be tested in a room adjacent to his ward, while the informant was seen in a separate appointment at home or at the research office. Most commonly, however, for the regular test, we saw the patient and informant at the same time and place. In all such instances it was essential to have them out of earshot of each other as long as either was being tested, to preserve the independence of each party's report.

For a quite small minority of evaluations, the examiner met the participants neither at the hospital nor at home, but "elsewhere." This ensued from our policy of going out of our way to meet the participants' convenience—an antidote to the ever-present threat of massive attrition. Thus we conducted a few sessions at outpatient clinics other than the one at Spring Grove in conjunction with patient's treatment visits; other participants were seen at their own proprietary places of business, and others at the Day Center on the hospital grounds.

Even more sensitive than the problem of place was that of the informant. Having taken pains to enlist the most suitable informant available for Test 1, we faced thereafter the issue of informant continuity. What if this same person should become unavailable for later tests? Conservative classical test theory would forbid substitutions as violations of month-to-month comparability of measurements. But such purity was neither possible in practice nor uniformly desirable in principle—when principle included ordinary considerations of social ecology. The practical impossibility is self-evident; an informant might die, or his divorce from the patient might just as irretrievably remove him from the running. The cardinal point was that the informant *for each session* should be a "significant other" in the patient's *current* environment—specifically, that person among any number of available relatives and friends who, at that particular time, was most knowledgeable about the patient's behavior. Whenever the patient's environmental flux shifted the identity of this person, as when one patient moved to a different household, we sought to shift informants accordingly. Fortunately in most instances, as would be expected, this policy accorded with the participants' own convenience and propensities. Once or twice, however, it was impossible to recruit any adequate informant because of the patient's "lone wolf" pattern of alienation from humanity at large.

Another locus of the continuity-*vs.*-change issue was the examiner. Optimally, the same examiner would test all patients and all informants throughout the entire study so as to prevent any spurious variance whatever in scores due to examiner differences. Here we took no exception in principle to orthodox psychometrics, but realities ruled otherwise, as is true even in many controlled experiments. More than one examiner was needed to carry the caseload; and some examiners might (and did, during 29 months of testing) resign before all of the patients they were following could complete the study year. Apart from these prime reasons for changes, there were few occasions for lapses in examiner constancy. One such temporary condition was minor reorganization of staff functions as the study got under way. Another, sporadic, was the unavoidable absence of a given "constant" examiner on vacation, illness, or testing of another case. Finally, to complete the list, there were two other circumstances, both extremely rare. The first had to do with a few single sessions in which the patient and informant had to be tested by two different examiners. This would happen, for example, when a patient was tested at our office while his informant preferred to be seen at home, and the same examiner could not cover both appointments. The other rare circumstance was when after staff discussion we felt that resistance to follow-up was attributable to personal incompatibility of examiner and participant; this called for a change of examiner in the hope of mitigating the resistance.

## EVALUATION TECHNIQUES: BACKGROUND DATA

For each patient, including nonparticipants, background data were compiled from hospital records. This information fell into three categories:

*1. Demographic.* Date of birth; age at time of leaving hospital; sex; race; marital status; number of children born to patient; religious preference; years of education completed; most recent occupation—major group as listed in the *Dictionary of Occupational Titles* (Division of Occupational Analysis, United States Employment Service, 1949, p. ix).

*2. Clinical: Last Pre-study Hospitalization.* Final diagnosis when leaving hospital; dates of admission and release; number of months hospitalized; type of release; whether or not drug treatment was received at any time.

*3. Clinical: Earlier Hospitalizations.* Number of hospitalizations; total number of years hospitalized, to nearest whole number. The last pre-study hospitalization was not included in either of these counts.

Our project goals placed only a minor emphasis on predicting posthospital adjustment from pre-release data; otherwise the above list might well have contained numerous additional clinical and psychometric variables. Instead, our background items were intended mainly as aids for defining the sample, interpreting results, and comparing our findings with those of other posthospital studies.

## EVALUATION TECHNIQUES: KATZ ADJUSTMENT SCALES

The main instrument used for the monthly posthospital evaluations of community adjustment was the Katz Adjustment Scales (KAS). Their content is shown in Appendixes E and F, and special procedures in administering them are covered in Appendix G. Katz and Lyerly (1963) have presented in detail the scales' rationale and description, together with early work on scale development and validation. Grossly, the KAS is an objectively scored multiple-choice pencil-and-paper questionnaire. One booklet is for use by the patient; it comprises five "forms," S1 through S5. A second booklet, for independent use by a relative or other informant with close personal knowledge of the patient, also comprises five forms (R1 through R5), of which the last four are quite similar or identical to the corresponding S Forms. As the authors have stated, "the major characteristics of the scales are their reliance on both the patient and a relative in measuring social behavior, the use of a relative as a direct reporter, and the establishment of his reliability in describing patient behavior" (Katz and Lyerly, 1963).

Six measures of community adjustment are derived from the patient forms (Table I-1) and 18 from the informant forms (Table I-2). As is evident from Table I-2, Form R1 contains 41 items which were not scored for our evaluations. These items had been used in earlier research and were retained for their potential usefulness in later work.[3]

To oversimplify considerably the KAS authors' methodology, the following constructs are embodied principally though not exclusively in the indicated KAS forms:

Clinical adjustment: S1, R1
Adequate social functioning: S2, S4, R2, R4
Social adjustment: R2 cf. R3; R5
Personal adjustment: S1; S2 cf. S3; S5
Social behavior: R1

Forms S3 and R3, Level of Expectations for patient and informant, are not per se directly affiliated with any of the above constructs. They do provide, however, "satisfaction" scores by enabling us to compare the reported *expectations* with reported

*Table I-1. Measures Obtained from Katz Adjustment Scales, Patient Forms*

| Form No. | Title | No. of Items |
|---|---|---|
| S1 | Symptom Discomfort | 55 |
| S2 | Level of Performance of Socially-Expected Activities | 16 |
| S3 | Level of Expectations | 16 |
| S2, S3 | Level of Satisfaction with Performance of Socially-Expected Activities[a] | 16 + 16 |
| RS4 | Level of Free-Time Activities | 22[b] |
| S5 | Level of Satisfaction with Free-Time Activities | 22[b] |

[a]A discrepancy measure, based on item-for-item comparison of Forms S2 and S3.

[b]A 23rd item, "Other (what?)__________," was also used, for write-ins, but was not scored.

[3]Detailed procedure for scoring the KAS is not presented in this volume. In scoring as well as in content, our version of the KAS (Appendixes E and F) differed slightly from the scoring and content set forth in the original report (Katz and Lyerly, 1963). Later KAS usage, as of this writing, has entailed further minor modifications. Readers who desire current and complete information on the KAS for use in testing should write to the second author of this book.

*Table I-2. Measures Obtained from Katz Adjustment Scales, Informant Forms*

| Form No. (Cluster No.) | Title | No. of Items |
|---|---|---|
| R1 | Relative's Ratings of Patient Symptoms and Social Behavior:[a] | (127) |
| R1 (1) | Belligerence (28, 45, 50; II-38)[b] | 4 |
| R1 (2) | Verbal Expansiveness (II-24, -25, -30, -31, -43) | 5 |
| R1 (3) | Negativism (36, 37, 46, 47, 48, 51, 56, 59, 60) | 9 |
| R1 (4) | Helplessness (3, 74; II-17, II-18) | 4 |
| R1 (5) | Suspiciousness (40, 43; II-32, -33) | 4 |
| R1 (6) | Anxiety (18, 19, 23; II-36, -48, -50) | 6 |
| R1 (7) | Withdrawal and Retardation (8, 17, 70; II-1, -5, -9) | 6 |
| R1 (8) | General Psychopathology (5, 12, 30, 31, 32, 33, 34, 42, 44, 52, 55, 67, 71, 73; II-4, -15, -16, -19, -22, -23, -35, -44, -46, -52) | 24 |
| R1 (9) | Nervousness (20, 21, 22, 38) | 4 |
| R1 (10) | Confusion (II-10, -11, -13) | 3 |
| R1 (11) | Bizarreness (24, 25, 26; II-41, -49) | 5 |
| R1 (12) | Hyperactivity (6, 7, 13) | 3 |
| R1 (13) | Emotional Stability (39, 53, 54, 57, 58, 62, 63, 66, 75) | 9 |
| R2 | Level of Performance of Socially-Expected Activities | 16 |
| R3 | Level of Expectations | 16 |
| R2, R3 | Level of Satisfaction with Performance of Socially-Expected Activities[c] | 16 + 16 |
| RS4 | Level of Free-Time Activities | 22[d] |
| R5 | Level of Satisfaction with Free-Time Activities | 22[d] |

[a]Form R1 was not scored as a single scale. It yields 13 cluster scores titled as shown.

[b]Numbers following each cluster indicate the item numbers in Form R1 which compose the cluster. The prefix "II-" signifies that the item is found in Part II of Form R1.

[c]A discrepancy measure, based on item-for-item comparison of Forms R2 and R3.

[d]A 23rd item, "Other (what?)__________," was also used, for write-ins, but was not scored.

*performances* on the same social behavior items in Forms S2 and R2. This was the KAS authors' original intent for the S3 and R3 forms. Accordingly, at each administration of these subtests, we asked both respondents, patient and informant, to judge the patient's performance in the past month by what they could recall they had expected at the start of his posthospital year. As Katz and Lyerly (1963) have noted, we thus registered the respondent's "retrospective level of aspiration," while the indirect use of the responses in obtaining the discrepancy score (expectations cf. performances) ruled out any need to assume that the report of expectations was either accurate or nonfluctuating. We did, nevertheless, also score S3 and R3 expectations as separate measures, for whatever value they might have as indexes of the patient's self-perception and the informant's perception of the patient. There was, of course, still another kind of fluctuation possible for these measures in our study, apart from retrospective error. If the newly released patient had been expected (or had expected himself) to improve throughout the year—or to worsen or follow any course other than a level one—then the successive monthly expectations scores would fluctuate accordingly to the extent that they were valid.

## EVALUATION TECHNIQUES: LIFE-SITUATION INTERVIEWS

Immediately after completing the KAS, each patient and informant underwent a structured interview with the examiner. Independence of the two reports was preserved as for the KAS. Patient and informant interviews were similar but not identical. Their purpose was to gather largely factual information which would picture the patient's ongoing life situation in some of its significant demographic, social, and clinical aspects. Some of this information supplemented the evaluative function of the KAS, while other items provided interpretive background for the evaluation measures.

Appendixes H and I present the patient and informant interview items, except for the special section on Recent and Current Life Stresses which is shown separately in Appendix J. In designing the Life Stresses section we drew upon a much more complex inventory of "situational variables" by Sargent, Modlin, Faris, and Voth (1958). Our stress inquiry was devised to explore the function of environmental stress in the course of mental illness. As a measurement technique it was both novel and provisional; therefore we have analyzed preliminary results from early and incomplete data collected for the present study (Michaux, Gansereit, McCabe, and Kurland, 1967). The analysis indicated that a stress inquiry was potentially useful and meaningful as a research and clinical tool.

## EVALUATION TECHNIQUES: REHOSPITALIZATION RECORDS

Rehospitalization *vs.* remaining in the community was a major dependent variable. For the follow-up year as a whole, records were kept on total number of rehospitalizations per patient and total days rehospitalized. For the monthly evaluations, each patient's hospital status was noted as "in" or "out"; "in" was defined as being rehospitalized for one or more days during the month.

Inasmuch as hospital treatment was not being evaluated, we recorded only one other datum on inpatient experience. Whenever a rehospitalization was terminated by release during the study year, we noted whether or not it had included drug therapy. In the entire study there was only one terminated rehospitalization during which the patient did *not* have any drug therapy; therefore this variable has been dropped from further analysis.

## *OBTAINED AND MISSING DATA

A total of 218 qualified ex-patients were selected and asked to take Test 1. Seventy-nine of these (36.2 per cent) failed to complete the first of 12 possible evaluations, thus automatically becoming nonparticipants with no tests completed (Figure I-1, box C). This was the point of peak attrition; of the 139 patients who did complete Test 1, only 48 (22.0 per cent of 218) ended the study with an appreciable number of monthly tests unjustifiably missed, i.e., for any reason except rehospitalization. From the standpoint of personal commitment to participating in the study, it appears that completion of Test 1 was the major hurdle, where most of the seriously refractory cases were eliminated.

The 36.2 per cent attrition for Test 1 seems high in some respects. It does not appear deviantly so, however, when one considers three factors involved in our recruiting for Test 1:

*1. Dynamics.* A candidate might understandably react aversively when, having freshly left the hospital and returned home, he was contacted by persons not previously known to him and asked to report on his condition.

*2. Limits of manpower and recruiting time.* While new patients were being recruited, the project staff was also obliged to maintain the rather complex network of monthly appointments and tests for patients already under study. Moreover, the total time available for recruiting each candidate was, so to speak, constrained at both ends. At the starting end, there was the often unavoidable delay of as much as 20 posthospital days to obtain all necessary screening information from the final hospital-discharge notes. This left about three weeks for the eligible patient to be located and contacted, and for him and his informant to be prevailed upon to take Test 1 not later than the 40th posthospital day.

*3. Long-range motivational and logistical considerations.* There was considerable interaction between this factor and *2.* For patients and/or informants who proved difficult to recruit, it was only sensible to consider their specific participation difficulties from the standpoint of prognosis for completing Tests 2 through 12, when deciding just how much staff effort to invest in obtaining Test 1. In this way, the chances of missed tests later in the series could be lessened. This principle, however, was used with restraint, even though replacements were amply available; to have used it freely would have aggravated the risk of sampling bias.

Among the 139 patients who with their informants took the first test, there was considerable variation in degree of further cooperation with the study as the year progressed. To organize and conserve as much obtained data as possible, we classified each case, after the year had ended, in one of three groups: complete, semicomplete, or incomplete. Table I-3 gives the essential criteria for the groupings and shows how the 139 cases were distributed. Sex distributions within the three groups are presented in Appendix N, Table N-9.

Criteria for the complete category were such that scores for the occasional missed tests, when required for a particular data analysis, could be estimated and inserted in the monthly series without transgressing statistical tolerance limits. The intermediate semicomplete group had as its main asset the completion of initial and final tests, but was limited by much missing data for the other 10 months. By pooling complete and semicomplete cases, we had available up to 120 cases for those analyses involving Adjustment

*Table I-3. Classification of Participants by Amount of Data Obtained*

| Classification | $N$ | Per Cent | Criteria |
|---|---|---|---|
| Complete | 91 | 65.5 | Tests 1 and 12 completed<br>At least 8 tests completed for Months 2 through 11 |
| Semicomplete | 29 | 20.9 | Tests 1 and 12 completed<br>Not more than 7 tests completed for Months 2 through 11 |
| Incomplete | 19 | 13.7 | Test 1 completed<br>Test 12 missed |
| All Participants | 139 | ≑100.0 | Minimum: Test 1 completed. |

and Life Situation data only for Months 1 and 12. The smaller incomplete group could be used when analysis was confined to Month-1 test data; in these instances, the incompletes could be pooled with all other cases for a maximum total $N$ of 139.

Detailed statistics on the net yield of usable data are presented in Table I-4. For the total sample, illegitimately missed tests outnumbered those legitimately missed by two to one; in the "complete" group alone, however, the rate of illegitimate misses was, as arranged, very low. Monthly coverage of the complete group's in-community time throughout their study year was thus virtually uninterrupted. An average of 9.9 monthly evaluations per patient (899 evaluations divided by 91 cases) were actually obtained in this group, while the semicompletes averaged only 3.9 sessions per case and the incompletes 3.2.

Figure I-2 depicts the monthly course of data attrition. For the semicompletes and incompletes, the rates differ little except at Month 12, the decisive choice-point for these two classifications.

## *VARIABLES IN THE TESTING SITUATION

The testing situation included five noteworthy variables which by nature eluded maximum control: the time interval between monthly appointments, the place of testing, identity of the examiner, identity of the informant, and proximity of patient and in-

*Table I-4. Tests Obtained, Illegitimately Missed, and Legitimately Missed: Entire Project*

| Testing Outcome | Complete | | Semicomplete | | Incomplete | | Total | |
|---|---|---|---|---|---|---|---|---|
| | *N* | Per Cent | *N* | Per Cent | *N* | Per Cent | *N* | Per Cent |
| Obtained: | | | | | | | | |
| Patient | 899 | 82.3 | 114 | 32.8 | 62 | 27.2 | 1075 | 64.4 |
| Informant | 900 | 82.4 | 103 | 29.6 | 59 | 25.9 | 1062 | 63.7 |
| Illegitimately missed: | | | | | | | | |
| Patient | 33 | 3.0 | 216 | 62.1 | 150 | 65.8 | 399 | 23.9 |
| Informant | 32 | 2.9 | 227 | 65.2 | 153 | 67.1 | 412 | 24.7 |
| Legitimately missed:[a] | | | | | | | | |
| Patient | 160 | 14.7 | 18 | 5.2 | 16 | 7.0 | 194 | 11.6 |
| Informant | 160 | 14.7 | 18 | 5.2 | 16 | 7.0 | 194 | 11.6 |
| Total: | | | | | | | | |
| Patient | 1092 | 100.0 | 348 | ÷100.0 | 228 | 100.0 | 1668 | ÷100.0 |
| Informant | 1092 | 100.0 | 348 | 100.0 | 228 | 100.0 | 1668 | 100.0 |

[a]Limited to rehospitalization with one exception: in the "incomplete" group, one patient was deceased at Months 11 and 12.

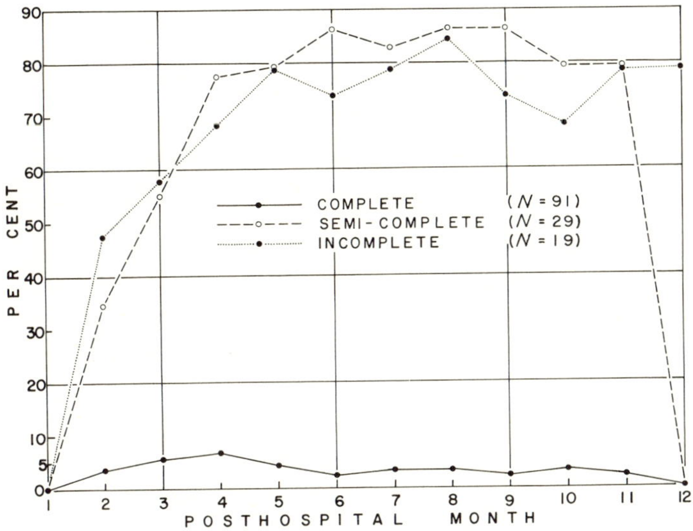


Figure I-2. Monthly incidence of illegitimately missed patient tests in the three data groups. All per cents are based on total *N*s as shown. Incidence lines for informant tests (not shown) would differ slightly from the patient lines because not quite all missed tests were missed by both respondents. (At Month 12, all 19 of the incompletes actually had missing data, but only 79 per cent (15 cases) are so plotted; the remaining four cases were in the hospital at Month 12, had missed the relapse test during an earlier month, and, in accord with our rule, became special cases whose rehospitalization status did not excuse their missed Test 12.)

formant to each other in their daily living. Appendix K presents descriptive data on each variable.

Throughout every patient's study year we sought to prevent impropriety and undue fluctuation with reference to each of these factors. While this is the most that one can do in a longitudinal field study with volunteer subjects, it is also the least that is needed to avoid inordinate error variance. Given the project's design and working conditions, we are satisfied that the results of these efforts were close to the optimum attainable.

Variation in the identity of the examiner, as opposed to the ideal of the same single examiner for all subjects and all repeated measurements, was the most noticeable situational irregularity (Appendix K: Tables K-5 and K-6). From the total pool of eight persons who served as examiners, two to three different individuals were needed to complete data collection for the average case.

The desirable interval of about 30 days between successive tests was approximated quite closely in three out of four instances, judging from a randomly selective compilation (Appendix K: Table K-1). The most frequent place of testing, as represented by Months 1, 6, and 12 combined, was the home of the patient and/or informant, where nearly half of the evaluations were conducted via examiner visits. The research office location was a close second in frequency, followed by a small minority of "all other" places (Appendix K: Tables K-2, K-3, and K-4).

It is difficult if not impossible, at least without intensive case study, to specify who is the best informant for a given patient. Our negotiable preference for spouse, parent, sibling, and so on, in that order, was based mainly on the obvious general clinical and social consideration of interpersonal closeness to the patient. Expectedly, this factor appears to have been positively correlated with availability and willingness to serve, for spouses predominated as informants, and frequencies for other informant-patient relationships followed quite closely our order of preference (Appendix K: Table K-8). Once an informant was enlisted, he tended not to withdraw from later evaulations unless the patient also withdrew. For the average patient, not more than two different persons served as informant throughout testing; for the majority, not more than one (Appendix K: Table K-7). Only a small proportion of informants were living apart from the patients (Appendix K: Table K-9). All in all, then, the informant situation deviated little from optimum propriety and stability.

## SUMMARY

This study has sought to evaluate longitudinally, and more comprehensively than is usually the case, the posthospital adjustment of recently released psychiatric patients. It was also conceived as a trial demonstration of novel methods. A major novelty was our effort to evaluate each patient monthly for one year, except during time lost by rehospitalization.

A random sample of eligible patients was drawn from the day-to-day release records of Spring Grove State Hospital, one of four large public psychiatric institutions serving the state of Maryland

and located near the City of Baltimore. The sample comprised adult white ex-patients of both sexes who had either been directly discharged or placed on long-term convalescent leave. Mental defectives and cases with organic central nervous system disorders were excluded; to be eligible diagnostically, a patient could have any functional psychiatric diagnosis except alcoholism or drug addiction. It was necessary, largely for practical reasons, to debar from the sample all patients who became rehospitalized within the first 20 days after having left Spring Grove.

Voluntary participation in the study was sought from a total of 218 patients identified as eligible. Enough data were obtained on 139 patients to include them in analyses to be presented. When all subjects had finished the posthospital study year, there were 91 cases classifiable as "complete," 29 as "semicomplete," and 19 as "incomplete."

Demographic and clinical background data were compiled from hospital records. All 139 patients in the study sample completed the Month-1 baseline evaluation; those who failed to do so were automatically dropped. A slightly less stringent premium was placed on completion of the final evaluation at Month 12. If a patient became rehospitalized during his study year, a special "relapse" evaluation was conducted in order to cover whatever time had elapsed since he had completed his last regular monthly evaluation; if the same patient subsequently returned to the community, the regular monthly schedule was resumed.

We obtained data not only from the patient himself but also from a qualified informant, usually a close relative. The main assessment instrument was the Katz Adjustment Scales (KAS), the use of which was another aspect of our trial demonstration of new methods. After completing the KAS, each respondent also underwent a Life Situation Interview, aimed at collecting relevant supplemental information and containing a newly developed short scale for measuring environmental stress.

Chapter II

# Description of the Sample

Before discussing our results, let us make explicit eight self-imposed rules of thumb which, if left unstated, could puzzle or perplex the reader. They apply to the entire body of findings throughout the report and they concern:

*1. Variations in size of groups analyzed.* In dealing with each question to be answered by statistical analysis, our strategy has been generally to use all available case data applicable to that particular question. The amount of available data, however, will obviously vary from one analysis to another. For example, rehospitalized patients were legitimately unavailable for monthly evaluations of in-community adjustment; and the "incomplete" group, which by definition missed Test 12, is thereby absent from Month-12 analyses. Additionally, for those analyses involving Months 2 through 11, we have not used the few tests taken by patients classified semicomplete and incomplete (Figure I-2), for their inclusion would have occasioned still further (monthly) undesirable variations in sample composition.

*2. Minimal use of control-variable analyses.* Except in a few special instances, we have not undertaken to control independent variables when formulating data analyses. The study's prime intent has been to delineate grossly some of the major trends in posthospital adjustment which may merit further, more refined study.

Sex, for example, is often controlled in similar investigations, and properly so. Our decision not to analyze for males and females separately in this study was influenced though of course not compelled by the knowledge that, in our own data as well as in considerable earlier work which was known to us, sex differences on the KAS are negligible. With a sample as small as ours, to have undertaken such controls as a matter of general policy would have been to risk an infinite regress both of labor and of sample fractionation. Other field studies of mental disorder have failed to show consistent relationships of either age or sex to severity of illness (Dohrenwend and Dohrenwend, 1965).

*3. Significance tests: chi square unless noted.* Except where indicated, reported tests of significance are based on chi square, corrected for continuity as needed. When very small cell frequencies were encountered, we substituted for chi square the Fisher exact probability tests, using two-tailed $p$ values.

*4. Significance tests: usually two-tailed.* Wherever a choice has been possible between one- and two-tailed significance tests, we have favored the latter, except in a few instances where we have stated otherwise. In an exploratory field study like this one, with many variables to be traced across the board, alternatives seemed undesirable. To shuttle back and forth from one- to two-tailed tests would unduly complicate presentations of findings. Moreover, the hazardous ambiguities of one-tailed predictions are familiar alike to clinical-minded researchers and to research-minded clinicians. How safe is it to expect similar outcomes for acute and chronic illnesses? To achieve a salutary outcome, should a patient score favorably or unfavorably on a given predictor variable?

*5. Significance tests: attention to borderline results.* Many of our significance tests yielded borderline results ($p < .10$), or results approaching the borderline range ($p < .20$, etc.). In general, we have been strongly disinclined to ignore the reporting of such results, especially since a two-tailed test with $p < .10$ would, if considered as a one-tailed test, have $p < .05$. For each of our analyses, typically involving several variables each subjected separately to the same significance test, we have sought to present enough of the borderline and near-borderline results to be sure of salvaging any hypotheses which, in future studies with tighter controls, might yield results of definite significance both statistical and clinical.

*6. Adjustment variables: no factor-analytic treatment.* As will be seen, many of the adjustment variables which we tracked throughout the posthospital year exhibited high intercorrelations. We considered, but decided not to undertake, consolidation via factor analysis. Central to the decision was the concurrent developmental status of the KAS, which contained nearly all of our adjustment variables. In terms of further method development, there was need for additional knowledge of just how the separate KAS scales performed in assessing patients living at large in the community. A second and supporting consideration against KAS factor analysis was that factorial measures from other tests have not always excelled in posthospital predictions: the opposite was true, for example, in the work of Marks, Stauffacher, and Lyle (1963), who used the MMPI and the 16 PF test.

Apropos of this rule of thumb, we have used at certain junctures in the analysis a "global adjustment" score introduced later, based on empirically derived weightings of five of the KAS scores. We have limited its use to those instances where it seemed essential for answering certain questions; it is not included among our standard adjustment variables.

*7. Stress Index: dual treatment of raw data.* Information obtained by the Stress Inquiry (Appendix J) has been used under both of our major evaluation rubrics, "adjustment" and "life situation." Under "adjustment" we have analyzed parametrically the two Specific Stress Index scores, one from the patient's interview and one from the informant's interview. Under "life situation," we have nonparametrically analyzed each of the eight stress items, i.e., the two for general stress and the six for specific stress. The item-analysis approach, in particular as regards the six specific stress items, serves to identify sources of stress in terms of environmentally defined areas of the patient's experience. Throughout the report we use the term "stress index" to refer only to the Specific Stress Index, since we have left the very brief General Stress Index unscored except for the nonparametric item analyses.

*8. Percentages: whole numbers* vs. *decimalized.* Whenever a total $N$ is 100 or more, corresponding percentages are reported to one place beyond the decimal; when a total frequency is smaller than 100, percentages are rounded to whole numbers.

## BACKGROUND VARIABLES

The 139 patients who with suitable informants completed Test 1 constituted our total sample of participants. All patients were of the white race except for one American Indian male; all but three had received some form of drug treatment during the last pre-study hospitalization. Race and inpatient drug treatment (some *vs.* none) have therefore been eliminated from the variables to be studied.

Gross descriptive data for the remaining relevant demographic variables are presented in Table II-1. The participants' mean age was 41.1, S.D. 12.2. Their education averaged 10.4 years, S.D. 2.8. Among the 115 ever-married patients, the median number of children was 2.1 and the range was from 0 to 9 or more.

Three of the five relevant clinical background variables (Table II-2) pertain to psychiatric hospitalization. While one-fourth of the participants were first-admission patients, the sample as a whole had a median of 1.4 hospitalizations and 4.7 months' total inpatient time prior to the last pre-study admission. For the last hospitalization, immediately before starting our study, the median duration was 2.4 months.

Under "Final hospital diagnosis," one major eligible category, "psychophysiologic autonomic and visceral disorders," is not represented by any participant; this might have been expected, however, considering our limited sample size and the extremely low prevalence of this category in official statistics on the Spring Grove ex-patient population (U.S. Department of Health, Education, and Welfare, and Maryland State Department of Mental Hygiene, 1964). Appendix L provides detailed information on specific diagnoses.

Condensing these descriptive data into a composite picture, we can visualize the typical participant as a white 41-year-old housewife who had left Spring Grove with a schizophrenic diagnosis. She was of the Protestant faith, had not finished high school, and had never been gainfully employed. The care of two children was

*Table II-1. Demographic Background Variables: Distributions for Participants (N = 139)*

| Variable | | N | Per Cent |
|---|---|---|---|
| Age: | 18 to 29 | 29 | 20.9 |
| | 30 to 39 | 32 | 23.0 |
| | 40 to 49 | 38 | 27.3 |
| | 50 to 59 | 31 | 22.3 |
| | 60 to 69 | 8 | 5.8 |
| | 70 to 74 | 1 | 0.7 |
| Sex: | Male | 44 | 31.7 |
| | Female | 95 | 68.3 |
| Marital status: | Single | 24 | 17.3 |
| | Married | 87 | 62.6 |
| | Widowed | 5 | 3.6 |
| | Separated | 17 | 12.2 |
| | Divorced | 6 | 4.3 |
| Number of children: | None | 36 | 25.9 |
| | One | 23 | 16.5 |
| | Two | 36 | 25.9 |
| | Three or four | 36 | 25.9 |
| | Five or more | 8 | 5.8 |
| Religion: | Catholic | 47 | 33.8 |
| | Protestant | 85 | 61.2 |
| | Jewish | 6 | 4.3 |
| | None | 1 | 0.7 |
| Years of education: | 4 to 8 | 40 | 28.8 |
| | 9 to 11 | 36 | 25.9 |
| | 12 | 44 | 31.7 |
| | 13 to 19 | 19 | 13.7 |
| Occupation: | Never employed | 80 | 57.6 |
| | Professional and managerial | 8 | 5.8 |
| | Clerical and sales | 18 | 12.9 |
| | Service | 8 | 5.8 |
| | Agriculture, fishing, and forestry | 1 | 0.7 |
| | Skilled labor | 8 | 5.8 |
| | Semi-skilled labor | 9 | 6.5 |
| | Unskilled labor | 7 | 5.0 |

perhaps her prime social obligation. Her Spring Grove doctor had placed her on convalescent leave, thus keeping the door unlocked for rehospitalization.

## ADJUSTMENT AT MONTH 1

Table II-3 presents the earliest and most complete posthospital information obtained on the participants' in-community adjust-

*Table II-2. Clinical Background Variables: Distributions for Participants (N = 139)*

| Variable | *N* | Per Cent |
|---|---|---|
| No. of hospitalizations prior to last: | | |
| None (first admission) | 40 | 28.8 |
| One | 32 | 23.0 |
| Two or three | 28 | 20.1 |
| Four or five | 20 | 14.4 |
| Six or more | 19 | 13.7 |
| Years hospitalized prior to last admission: | | |
| None (first admission) | 40 | 28.8 |
| One-half or less | 34 | 24.5 |
| One | 31 | 22.3 |
| Two to fifteen | 27 | 19.4 |
| Unknown | 7 | 5.0 |
| Months hospitalized during last admission: | | |
| One or less | 37 | 26.6 |
| Two | 36 | 25.9 |
| Three | 24 | 17.3 |
| Four to six | 22 | 15.8 |
| Seven to seventy-five | 20 | 14.4 |
| Final hospital diagnosis: | | |
| Schizophrenic reaction (all types) | 76 | 54.7 |
| Psychoses other than schizophrenia | 28 | 20.1 |
| Psychoneurotic disorders | 24 | 17.3 |
| Personality disorders | 11 | 7.9 |
| Type of release from hospital: | | |
| Convalescent leave | 115 | 82.7 |
| Discharge with doctor's consent | 24 | 17.3 |

ment. Only at Month 1 were tests obtained on every single subject; at each of the succeeding 11 months some tests were missed illegitimately and/or because of rehospitalization. In the table we have listed the 24 KAS variables plus the two parametric stress variables: these 26 measures are to be treated as adjustment variables, in the standard sequence indicated, throughout the report. To identify them, we shall rely mainly on the symbols in the second column. All three of the footnoted procedures are also generally applicable and should be kept in mind continually by the reader. A final procedural arrangement has to do with the direction of scoring on the KAS scales. As indicated under "possible scores," *high* raw scores on adjustment variables are *unfavorable*, with five exceptions: on the following KAS scales *high scores are favorable:*

*Table II-3. Adjustment Variables: Descriptive Information and Status of Participants (N = 139) at Month 1*

| Scale: Title | Scale: Symbol[a] | Possible Scores: Best | Possible Scores: Worst | Participants at Month 1: Mean | Participants at Month 1: S.D. |
|---|---|---|---|---|---|
| KAS Patient Scales: | | | | | |
| Symptom Discomfort | *Sym* | 0[b] | 165[b] | 20.1 | 18.4 |
| Level of Performance of Socially-Expected Activities | *SEA-P* | 48 | 16 | 35.0 | 5.5 |
| Level of Expectations | *LOE-P* | 48 | 16 | 36.3 | 5.4 |
| Level of Satisfaction with Performance of Socially-Expected Activities | *SSA-P* | 0 | 67 | 7.9 | 8.4 |
| Level of Free-Time Activities | *FTA-P* | 22 | 66 | 48.0 | 5.8 |
| Level of Satisfaction with Free-Time Activities | *SFA-P* | 22 | 66 | 30.1 | 6.0 |
| KAS Informant Scales–Symptoms: | | | | | |
| Belligerence | *Bel* | 4 | 16 | 4.6 | 1.2 |
| Verbal Expansiveness | *Exp* | 5 | 20 | 6.3 | 2.2 |
| Negativism | *Neg* | 9 | 36 | 12.9 | 3.9 |
| Helplessness | *Hel* | 4 | 16 | 6.0 | 2.2 |
| Suspiciousness | *Sus* | 4 | 16 | 5.5 | 2.3 |
| Anxiety | *Anx* | 6 | 24 | 7.7 | 2.8 |
| Withdrawal and Retardation | *Wdl* | 6 | 24 | 10.0 | 3.2 |
| General Psychopathology | *Psy* | 24 | 96 | 36.1 | 10.2 |
| Nervousness | *Ner* | 4 | 16 | 7.9 | 2.8 |
| Confusion | *Con* | 3 | 12 | 3.5 | 1.4 |
| Bizarreness | *Biz* | 5 | 20 | 5.8 | 1.8 |
| Hyperactivity | *Hyp* | 3 | 12 | 4.9 | 1.7 |
| Emotional Stability | *Sta* | 36 | 9 | 28.8 | 5.8 |
| KAS Informant Scales–Social Behavior: | | | | | |
| Level of Performance of Socially-Expected Activities | *SEA-I* | 48 | 16 | 34.5 | 5.0 |
| Level of Expectations | *LOE-I* | 48 | 16 | 34.1 | 5.4 |
| Level of Satisfaction with Performance of Socially-Expected Activities | *SSA-I* | 0 | 67 | 6.2 | 6.8 |
| Level of Free-Time Activities | *FTA-I* | 22 | 66 | 49.2 | 5.4 |
| Level of Satisfaction with Free-Time Activities | *SFA-I* | 22 | 66 | 30.5 | 5.6 |
| Life Situation Interview–Stress Inquiry: | | | | | |
| Stress Index–Patient Interview | *Str-P* | 0[c] | 60[c] | 15.6 | 13.1 |
| Stress Index–Informant Interview | *Str-I* | 0[c] | 60[c] | 16.3 | 14.3 |

[a]The suffixes *-P* and *-I* indicate *patient* and *informant*, on those scales used in matching forms for both respondents.

[b]To reduce raw *Sym* scores to a size more convenient for data analysis, we subtracted 55 from each obtained score. In the original KAS scoring, the best and worst possible raw scores on *Sym* are 55 and 220.

[c]To augment raw scores on *Str-P* and *Str-I* to a more manageable size, we multiplied all obtained scores by 10. Thus the original raw-score range 0 . . . 6 becomes 0 . . . 60, and the seven possible scores are all multiples of 10.

*SEA–P* and *SEA–I* (Level of Performance of Socially-Expected Activities–patient and informant scales);

*LOE–P* and *LOE–I* (Level of Expectations–patient and informant scales); and

*Sta* (Emotional Stability–informant only).

In all presentations of results hereinafter (other than those exhibiting only raw-score workups) we have made appropriate reversals of score directions, etc., involving these five scales, so that a high score on any adjustment variable can be understood as unfavorable and vice versa. Reminders of these reversals and of unreversed raw scores are inserted in the text.

In themselves, the means and standard deviations in Table I-3 tell little clinically; they are useful primarily as baseline reference points against which other findings can be checked. We may note that for some variables the obtained scores tend to be concentrated toward the favorable or "perfect score" end of the continuum. Skewing is most pronounced in six of the 13 informant scales dealing with symptoms: *Bel* (Belligerence), *Exp* (Verbal Expansiveness), *Sus* (Suspiciousness), *Anx* (Anxiety), *Con* (Confusion), and *Biz* (Bizarreness). These scales seem to have registered comparatively very little in the way of disturbed adjustment in our patients shortly after they had left Spring Grove.

For the 18 KAS informant scales only, we had available other data from recent studies in Maryland which enabled us to place the Month-1 means in clinical perspective (Figure II-1). Graphic comparisons are thus possible with normals and with two groups of patients each at different levels of adjustment.

Grossly, our Spring Grove patients were not so well adjusted as the normals (represented by the grid-line at $T$ score = 50), but they were in considerably better condition than either the day-center patients or the about-to-be-hospitalized inpatients–the latter being the worst adjusted of all. If we think of the inpatient profile and the Spring Grove profile as pre- and post-treatment measures respectively, the differences suggest that hospitalization does help patients–though it would desecrate several canons of experimental design if we carried such an interpretation further

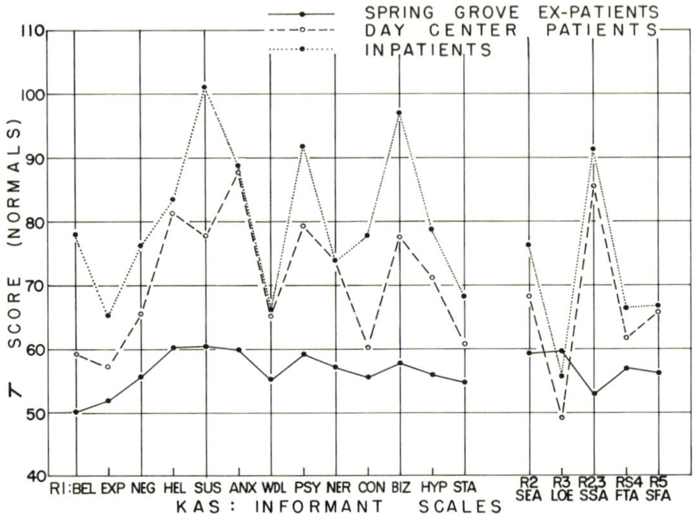


Figure II-1. Month-1 mean KAS informant scores of all participants ($N = 139$). Also plotted, for comparison, are means of 133 Baltimore Day Center patients and preadmission means of 42 inpatients at Springfield State Hospital, a Maryland institution similar to Spring Grove. The $T$ scale is based on scores of 450 representative normals in Carroll County, Maryland. To make high scores unfavorable on all KAS scales, direction is reversed for *Sta* (Stability), *SEA* (Socially-Expected Activities), and *LOE* (Level of Expectations). Data other than our own are from recent research by Gerard E. Hogarty and associates (Henri A. Lowery, personal communication, 1966).

than surmise. (Later evidence from our own study fails to support this conjecture.)

In discriminating among the three patient groups in Figure II-1, the most sensitive scales appear to be *Sus, Psy* (General Psychopathology), and *Biz.* These were among the six scales on which, interestingly enough, *both* of the non-Spring Grove groups had the highest elevations, the other three being *Hel* (helplessness), *Anx*, and *SSA* (Satisfaction with Socially-Expected Activities).

There is only one scale in the figure on which the ranking of the three patient group means deviates from the prevailing order: inpatients worst, Spring Grove patients best. That scale is *LOE*, where the informant was telling us to just what extent he expected the patient to be performing the socially-expected activities listed in the *SEA* scale. But here the three means are not comparable in the same sense as are the other means. The inpatient and day center informants were looking *ahead* and registering their expectations for patients who were *about to receive* treatment;[1] while the Spring Grove informants were looking *back* one month and telling what they had expected of patients who had *just finished* treatment. Nevertheless, it is instructive to consider the status of each of the three groups as regards (1) the difference between *SEA* and *LOE* and (2) the comparative height of *SSA*–the scale which in our sample reflects the degree of the informant's disappointment, based as it is on the composite discrepancies, item by item, between *SEA* and *LOE*. We can see that the inpatient and day center informants' expectations may well have been inordinately favorable–not only in these two respects, but also in that the treatment outcomes which they anticipated were better than the outcome actually achieved by the Spring Grove patients (*SEA*, solid line). If relatives are indeed vulnerable to disappointment with patients in this regard, their vulnerability is a starting point for specific mental health action in the community. In some groups of patients, it may behoove us to guide relatives toward realistic, less exalted expectations, thereby sparing them the kind of later dismay which could incur needless rehospitalization.

The single most striking feature of the Spring Grove group profile is that is appears so blandly flat and healthy in comparison with the elevation and jaggedness of the other two patient profiles. This came as a surprise to some colleagues who previewed the figure; others found it plausible. Just how disturbed should one have expected our patients to be at Month 1? We cannot confidently answer. To do so, one would have to be more definitive than realities allow in accounting for a number of conditions which could have influenced the KAS results. What might have been the psychometric implications of the various informants' relationships to the patients? In their KAS appraisals, to what extent were their subjective norms influenced by varying role expectations for individual patients (e.g., work *vs.* homemaking, housewife *vs.* unattached female)? How much weight, and in what direction, may have been carried by hospital standards for admission and discharge, as against informant standards for behavior?

[1]That is, the standard instructions for administering the KAS *LOE* scale were altered when the inpatient and day center informant data were collected.

Let us turn now from Figure II-1 to other aspects of Month-1 adjustment. We have already mentioned the tendency toward high intercorrelations among the 26 adjustment variables tabulated in Table II-3. Apposite statistics are recorded in Appendix M. In lieu of extensively discussing the intercorrelations, we have interpretively summarized them in the same appendix (Table M-2).

For five of our background variables, we calculated correlations with Month-1 scores on the 26 adjustment variables, $N = 139$.[2] Of the resulting 130 *r*s, only 13 were significant at or beyond the .05 level and all of these were of low to moderate magnitude. Results were as follows:[3]

*1. Age.* Advanced age was associated with favorable adjustment on four KAS measures: *SFA-P* (Satisfaction with Free-Time Activities—patient scale), $r = -.19$; *Hel*, $r = -.18$; *SSA-I*, $r = -.18$; *SFA-I*, $r = -.18$.

*2. Sex.* Point-biserial correlations were significant for five adjustment variables. Males tended toward poorer adjustment on *LOE-P*, -.18, and *FTA-P*, -.19. In contrast, females were slightly less favorably adjusted on *Bel*, .21; *Sus*, .20; and *Ner*, .19.

*3. Education.* None of the 26 *r*s was significant at the .05 level. One might have been inclined to expect otherwise: Education is a fairly sensitive index of socioeconomic status and the latter is now well known to be related to severity of mental illness (Hollingshead and Redlich, 1958; Dohrenwend and Dohrenwend, 1965). In our own findings, the lack of relationship between education and adjustment may be due to the relative homogeneity of our sample in both respects: Well-educated patients do not often enter public mental hospitals, and severely ill patients are rarely discharged from them. We have not included social class among variables to be studied, except indirectly, by way of the background variable "education." As we have just suggested, it seems unlikely that its inclusion would have been rewarding.

*4. Years hospitalized prior to last admission.* The only significant correlation was with *SEA-P*, .17: the longer the total prior

[2]Exception: $N = 132$ for "Years hospitalized prior to last admission" (unknown for seven cases).

[3]Positive and negative values of *r* have been reversed in some instances to homogenize raw-score directions: See text accompanying Table II-3.

hospitalization time, the poorer the performance of socially-expected activities during the first posthospital month.

5. *Months hospitalized during last admission.* Again, longer hospitalization was associated with unfavorable adjustment. Significant correlations were .31 with *SEA-P*, .23 with *LOE-P*, and .17 with *SSA-P.*

All of these correlations are of course interpretable as indexes of the usefulness of background variables in predicting early posthospital adjustment. In the present context, however, our interest is simply in their function as uncontrolled sampling variables. Later, in Chapter IV, all twelve background variables are tested as predictors of community adjustment.

A five-by-five matrix of intercorrelations among the same background variables yielded four significant *r*s and six nonsignificant. Sex was appreciably related to three of the other four variables: age (.23, $p < .01$, females older); years hospitalized prior to last admission (-.20, p. $< .05$, males hospitalized longer); and months hospitalized during last admission (-.22, *p.* $< .01$, males hospitalized longer). The only other significant correlation was that of .59 between years hospitalized prior to last admission and months hospitalized during last admission ($p < .001$). Age proved to be unrelated to the two length-of-hospitalization variables as well as to education. Education did not correlate significantly with any of the other items.

To consider "sex" more thoroughly and in relation to all of the other eleven background variables, we tested each of them dichotomously for differences between the 44 males and 95 females. Six of the eleven comparisons were nonsignificant, with *p* values from .30 for "religion" to .90 for "type of release." There were sizable sex differences on four of the six demographic variables plus only one of the five clinical variables (Table II-4). Females were older and, perhaps partly as a function thereof, more domestically settled. As was generally true in America during their youth, fewer of our females than of our males had ever entered any gainful employment.

The single tabulated clinical variable, "diagnosis," indicates that our males were typically schizophrenic and our nonschizophrenic psychotics were predominately female. The consistent lack of sig-

*Table II-4. Significant Sex Differences on Background Variables (Participants, N = 139)*

| Item | $p^a$ | Difference: Males | Difference: Females |
|---|---|---|---|
| Demographic variables: | | | |
| Age | .01 | Younger: M = 36.9, S.D. = 11.9 | Older: M = 43.0, S.D. = 11.8 |
| Marital status | .001 | More single (39 per cent), fewer married (41 per cent) | Fewer single (7 per cent), more married (73 per cent) |
| Number of children: | | | |
| All patients | .001 | Fewer children: Mdn = 0.6 | More children: Mdn = 2.1 |
| Ever-married patients ($N$ = 115) | .005 | Fewer children: Mdn = 1.6 | More children: Mdn = 2.2 |
| Occupation: | | | |
| All patients, including never-employed | .001 | Fewer never-employed (11 per cent) | More never-employed (79 per cent) |
| Patients with some work history ($N$ = 59) | .001 | More laborers (59 per cent) | Fewer laborers (10 per cent) |
| Clinical variable: | | | |
| Final hospital diagnosis | .025 | More schizophrenics (68 per cent), fewer other psychoses (7 per cent) | Fewer schizophrenics (48 per cent), more other psychoses (26 per cent) |

[a] All $p$ values based on $\chi^2$ except for Age ($t$, two-tailed test).

nificant or near-significant sex differences on the other four clinical background variables suggests that our males and females were essentially similar as regards hospitalization experience.

## LIFE SITUATION AT MONTH 1

To complete the description of our participants we now examine life situation, the third and final set of major variables. These are the data based on the patient and informant interviews which supplemented the KAS (Appendixes H, I, J). The sequence in which we deal with the variables here is standard for all subsequent analyses. Tabulations are again based on the earliest obtained reports, covering approximately the first 30 posthospital days.

The prevalent domestic scene to which the patients returned upon leaving Spring Grove was connubial (Table II-5). In the immediate family circle children figured more largely than did parents: More than half of the patients had at least one child in the home, while less than a fourth were living in homes presided over by parents. Only about half of the patients' mothers and fathers were still living.

Less than one patient in four had managed to start or resume work during the first month after returning home (Table II-6). (The unemployment rate for patients remaining in the community dropped to a low of 56 per cent at Month 8 and stood at 63 per cent at Month 12.) By the same token, at Month 1 only a small minority were making any substantial breadwinner contribution to family finances. In the "sheltered workshop" of the homemaker, however, nearly all of the females were undertaking partial or total responsibility.

Spring Grove State Hospital maintains an active and concerted aftercare program. Most patients who receive aftercare attend the Outpatient Clinic on the hospital grounds; some go to other state-operated clinics which may be located nearer their homes. Initiation of posthospital treatment immediately following release is the option of the doctor who discharges the patient. Psychotropic chemotherapy is the prime therapeutic tool. Simultaneously with leaving the hospital, a patient may be referred for his first out-

*Table II-5. Home and Family at Month 1 (Participants, N = 139)*

| Item | *N* | Per Cent |
|---|---|---|
| Type of home: | | |
| Conjugal | 87 | 62.6 |
| Parental | 32 | 23.0 |
| Other relative(s) | 12 | 8.6 |
| Solitary | 3 | 2.2 |
| All other | 5 | 3.6 |
| Own children in home: | | |
| None | 66 | 47.5 |
| One | 31 | 22.3 |
| Two | 23 | 16.5 |
| Three to six | 19 | 13.7 |
| Step-, in-law children in home: | | |
| None | 131 | 94.2 |
| One | 6 | 4.3 |
| Two | 2 | 1.4 |
| Own children away from home: | | |
| None | 78 | 56.1 |
| One | 33 | 23.7 |
| Two | 17 | 12.2 |
| Three to eight | 11 | 7.9 |
| Closest living relative: | | |
| Spouse | 103 | 74.1 |
| Parent | 29 | 20.9 |
| Child | 4 | 2.9 |
| Sibling | 3 | 2.2 |
| Mother living or deceased: | | |
| Living | 77 | 55.4 |
| Deceased | 62 | 44.6 |
| Father living or deceased: | | |
| Living | 62 | 44.6 |
| Deceased | 76 | 54.7 |
| Uncertain | 1 | 0.7 |

patient appointment, usually scheduled for about 30 days after his discharge; to maintain chemotherapy continuity, he may be provided with a temporary supply of posthospital medication. In the follow-up analyses we shall pay considerable attention to the patient's clinic attendance and to his reported consumption of drugs.

Four-fifths of the participants started the posthospital year with some form of aftercare (Table II-7). A large majority of those treated were seen at the Spring Grove clinic. Their outlook for future treatment portended little change in the Month-1 rate. (The

*Table II-6. Work and Homemaking at Month 1 (Participants, N = 139)*

| Item | Patient's Report | | Informant's Report | |
|---|---|---|---|---|
| | *N* | Per Cent | *N* | Per Cent |
| Employment duration: | | | | |
| No part of month | 109 | 78.4 | 109 | 78.4 |
| Half of month or less | 8 | 5.8 | 7 | 5.0 |
| More than half of month | 9 | 6.5 | 13 | 9.4 |
| All month | 13 | 9.4 | 10 | 7.2 |
| Busiest single work week:[a] | | | | |
| 1 . . . 17 hours | 3 | 10 | 4 | 14 |
| 18 . . . 34 hours | 5 | 17 | 3 | 10 |
| 35 + hours | 22 | 73 | 22 | 76 |
| Breadwinner contribution:[b] | | | | |
| No contribution | – | – | 85 | 66.4 |
| Minor contribution | – | – | 22 | 17.2 |
| About half of total | – | – | 8 | 6.2 |
| Major contribution | – | – | 4 | 3.1 |
| Sole breadwinner | – | – | 9 | 7.0 |
| Homemaker responsibility (females only): | | | | |
| No responsibility | 2 | 2 | 5 | 5 |
| One for self (solitary) | 2 | 2 | 2 | 2 |
| Shared responsibility | 37 | 39 | 35 | 37 |
| Sole responsibility | 54 | 57 | 53 | 56 |

[a]Employed patients only: $N = 30$. For informant's report, $N = 29$; in 1 case, informant did not know.

[b]Excluding 11 patients with no dependents to support. Item not used in patient interview.

*Table II-7. Outpatient Treatment at Month 1 (Participants, N = 139)*

| Item | *N* | Per Cent |
|---|---|---|
| Where received: | | |
| Nowhere (not in treatment) | 26 | 18.7 |
| Spring Grove Outpatient Clinic | 79 | 56.8 |
| Public clinic other than Spring Grove | 10 | 7.2 |
| Private psychiatrist | 8 | 5.8 |
| Private physician other than psychiatrist | 7 | 5.0 |
| All other | 9 | 6.5 |
| Outlook for future treatment: | | |
| No plan to continue or start[a] | 29 | 20.9 |
| Plan to continue or start[b] | 110 | 79.1 |

[a]If in treatment, would not be continuing; if not in treatment, would not be starting.

[b]If in treatment, would continue so; if not in treatment, would soon start.

actual untreated rate, reading 18.7 per cent at Month 1, subsequently fluctuated between a low of 18 per cent at Month 2 and a high of 28 per cent at Months 7 and 12.)

Table II-8 shows that the typical participant had a drug prescribed throughout all of Month 1, used it throughout the month,[4] and observed the prescribed daily dosage. We have heard such patients proclaim their reliance on the drug as a talisman for avoiding rehospitalization. For others, perhaps not so many, side effects (either verifiable or unverifiable) lend a dysphoric negative valence to medication.

*Table II-8. Drug Treatment at Month 1 (Participants, N = 139)*

| Item | Patient's Report | | Informant's Report | |
|---|---|---|---|---|
| | *N* | Per Cent | *N* | Per Cent |
| How long prescribed: | | | | |
| No part of month | 19 | 13.7 | 20 | 14.4 |
| Half of month or less | 5 | 3.6 | 2 | 1.4 |
| More than half of month | 5 | 3.6 | 3 | 2.2 |
| All of month | 110 | 79.1 | 111 | 79.9 |
| Unknown (informant only) | – | – | 3 | 2.2 |
| How long used:[a] | | | | |
| No part of time prescribed | 4 | 3.3 | 2 | 1.7 |
| Up to half of time prescribed | 3 | 2.5 | 7 | 6.0 |
| More than half of time prescribed | 14 | 11.7 | 9 | 7.8 |
| All of time prescribed[b] | 99 | 82.5 | 94 | 81.0 |
| Unknown (informant only) | – | – | 4 | 3.4 |
| Typical daily consumption:[a] | | | | |
| None | 4 | 3.3 | 2 | 1.7 |
| Up to half of prescribed dosage | 2 | 1.7 | 3 | 2.6 |
| More than half of prescribed dosage | 8 | 6.7 | 8 | 6.9 |
| All of prescribed dosage[c] | 106 | 88.3 | 93 | 80.2 |
| Unknown (informant only) | – | – | 10 | 8.6 |

[a]Data limited to patients who had drug prescribed: *N* = 120 for patient's report, 116 for informant's.

[b]Includes 1 case who used drug "Longer than time prescribed"–informant's report only.

[c]Includes 4 reports of "More than prescribed dosage": 1 from a patient, 3 from informants.

[4]Patients' oral reports of their own drug consumption, such as are represented in these data, have been found valid enough to be useful despite some inaccuracy. By carefully checking Baltimore outpatients' interview reports against pill counts, Park and Lipman (1964) ascertained that the major source of inaccuracy was the patient's tendency to report having taken all of the prescribed dosage when actually he had taken less. We know of no findings on the veridicality of informants' reports on drug consumption.

The treatment situation at Month 1, however it may have changed subsequently, was our subjects' posthospital heritage. As such, it merits closer inspection than we shall give it later in the year. Did participants receive any treatments other than drugs? If so, what were they, and what were the combinations when a given patient had more than one form of treatment? When drugs were prescribed, exactly which ones were chosen? Answers from patients' reports are compiled in Tables II-9 and II-10. From Table II-9 it is seen that more than half of the numerous drug-treated patients also received some other form of therapy—usually individual psychotherapy.[5] Patients who were not on drugs often went untreated.

*Table II-9. Type of Treatment Received at Month 1 (Participants, N = 139)*

| Type of Treatment | *N* | Per Cent |
|---|---|---|
| Sole treatment: | | |
| Drug(s) | 53 | 38.1 |
| Individual psychotherapy | 5 | 3.6 |
| Drug(s) combined with: | | |
| Individual psychotherapy only | 57 | 41.0 |
| Individual psychotherapy plus other(s)[a] | 6 | 4.3 |
| Other(s)[b] | 4 | 2.9 |
| Combined treatment without drug[c] | 1 | 0.7 |
| None (untreated) | 13 | 9.4 |
| Total | 139 | 100.0 |

[a]Group psychotherapy (4 cases); group psychotherapy plus occupational therapy (1); social casework (1).

[b]Group psychotherapy (3 cases), public health nurse home visits (1).

[c]Group psychotherapy plus Day Center attendance.

In psychiatric settings not rich in manpower, fees, or funds, chemotherapy is almost inevitably the modern treatment of choice. Nevertheless, the treatment approach to our patients was obviously not monolithic, and such diversity as is shown in Table

[5]We defined individual psychotherapy broadly so that it included (but was not limited to) interviewing lasting at least 10 minutes—provided the patient could report to us that it contained some effort to counsel or help him, i.e., was not intended merely to monitor his condition.

II-9 quite likely reflects serious clinical effort to fit the treatment to the individual patient.

In the total group of 19 patients who had no drug prescribed, only six, or 32 per cent, received any form of non-drug treatment. In contrast, among the 120 drug-treated patients, 67, (55.8 per cent) also received nonmedicinal therapy. This differential, significant at the .05 level ($\chi^2 = 3.87$), appears to be weighted paradoxically in the direction opposite to what one would expect—until we consider that for drug-treated patients the typical "other" treatment was very brief psychotherapy aimed at placing chemotherapy in meaningful clinical perspective.

*Table II-10. Psychiatric Drugs Prescribed at Month 1 (Participants, N = 139)*

| Prescribed Drug(s) | *N* | Per Cent |
|---|---|---|
| Chlorpromazine | 20 | 14.4 |
| Perphenazine | 13 | 9.4 |
| Thioridazine | 12 | 8.6 |
| Trifluoperazine | 9 | 6.5 |
| Chlordiazepoxide | 4 | 2.9 |
| Imipramine | 3 | 2.2 |
| Amitriptyline | 2 | 1.4 |
| Chlorprothixine | 2 | 1.4 |
| Two drugs concurrent[a] | 24 | 17.3 |
| Three drugs concurrent[b] | 4 | 2.9 |
| Unidentified drug(s) | 27 | 19.4 |
| None | 19 | 13.7 |
| Total | 139 | ≑100.0 |

[a]Paired drugs, in order of decreasing frequency, were: imipramine, trifluoperazine, thioridazine, chlorpromazine, amitriptyline, perphenazine, benztropin, chlordiazepoxide, phenobarbital, and secobarbital.

[b]Drugs prescribed concurrently in groups of three were: biperidin, chlorpromazine, imipramine, trifluoperazine, barbital, diphenylhydantoin, phenobarbital, and thioridazine.

Diversity characterized not only the type of aftercare treatment received but also the choice of drug to be prescribed (Table II-10). Antipsychotic drugs (chlorpromazine, perphenazine, thioridazine, trifluoperazine, chlorprothixine) were prescribed for 56 of the 65 patients who received single drugs of known identity. Five patients received an antidepressant (imipramine, amitriptyline) and four received an anti-anxiety compound (chlordiazepoxide).

Two other life situation variables pertaining to treatment have been excluded from all data analysis and are mentioned here only in passing. Although we tracked both items throughout the post-hospital year, distributions proved massivcly skewed and hence not potentially informative. (1) Very few patients reported having received any *secondary* psychiatric outpatient treatment[6]–viz., at a facility different from their primary one–at any time. At Month 1, 93.5 per cent of the 139 participants had no secondary treatment; at no later month did the figure drop below 84 per cent (Month 8) or exceed 94 per cent (Month 12). Throughout the year the favorite source of secondary psychiatric treatment was a private nonpsychiatric physician; this source was used by as many as 10 patients at Month 7 and by as few as 2 at Month 4. (2) *Tertiary* psychiatric outpatient treatment was received by not more than two patients during any of the 12 months.

As previously explained, the stress inquiry data are to be dealt with both by parametric scale analysis (Table II-3) and by non-parametric item analysis (Table II-11). The two general stress items are to be covered only by the latter procedure. Each percentage in Table II-11 indicates the proportion of patients "in

*Table II-11. Environmental Stresses at Month 1 (Participants, N = 139)*

| Item | Patient's Report | | Informant's Report | |
|---|---|---|---|---|
| | *N* | Per Cent[a] | *N* | Per Cent[a] |
| General stress: | | | | |
| *No* "Good" event during month | 65 | 46.8 | 68 | 48.9 |
| *Some* "Bad" event(s) during month | 50 | 36.0 | 54 | 38.8 |
| Specific stress experienced during month: | | | | |
| Interpersonal | 46 | 33.1 | 53 | 38.1 |
| Marital and sexual | 30 | 21.6 | 35 | 25.2 |
| Economic and domestic | 41 | 29.5 | 47 | 33.8 |
| Occupational | 44 | 31.7 | 44 | 31.7 |
| Social and recreational | 14 | 10.1 | 10 | 7.2 |
| Physical health | 42 | 30.2 | 37 | 26.6 |

[a]Each item is based on an interview question answered "Yes" or "No"; each per cent covers only one sector of the response dichotomy. See Appendix J for question wordings and for procedures to avoid topical overlap among Specific stress items.

[6]For main, secondary, and tertiary outpatient psychiatric treatment, the literal content of the data is shown in Appendix H, items 1, 2, and 3.

trouble" on a given item; in handling them thus, we always have to reverse the tabulation for the first item, where the respondent was asked if anything good had happened; here we tabulate the "no" answers, while "yes" answers are counted for the remaining seven items. (The informant is reporting not on his own stresses but on his observations of those experienced by the patient.)

None of the eight items was trouble-free at Month 1. The two general items polled more positive answers than did any of the specific items—more or less inevitably so in the case of "bad" event(s), as this question interlocks with all of the specific items (Appendix J). The disadvantage of the general items is their informational nonspecificity; their advantage is their open-ended dragnet and pump-priming function. By the gross psychometric consideration of discriminating power, all eight of the items in this provisional interview technique promised to be useful, with the possible exception of "social and recreational." Here the low positive yields of 10.1 and 7.2 per cent may reflect the circumscribed civic and leisure life associated with low socioeconomic status.

## *SAMPLING BIAS

The study's architectonics contained a liberal share of loopholes for sampling bias which by now are largely self-evident to the reader. This section reports our efforts to assay, loophole by loophole, just how much bias did infiltrate. Admittedly, we could have designed a more bias-proof investigation from the start; but we preferred not to compromise, as would have been imperative, our interest in the testing of new methods.

Does our sample adequately represent the Spring Grove ex-patient reference population as defined by our criteria? The answer is a qualified yes. Overall results of our sampling-bias analyses show that, while sampling was not flawless, it was not so aberrant that we must write off our results as clinically and scientifically meaningless; and further, that the warpings in our data are discernible and specifiable enough to be used as corrective guidelines in interpretation.

We shall deal with the question of sampling bias at four discrete levels and in the following sequence: (1) Insofar as direct comparison is practicable, how similar are our participants to the concurrent reference population of Spring Grove ex-patients? (2) To what degree do the 139 participants differ from the 79 equally eligible nonparticipants? (3) Many analyses were of necessity limited to the 91 complete cases; how does this particular subgroup compare with the nonparticipants? (4) Within the total participant group, what sort of bias was associated with missed tests (Figure I-2) as reflected by differences among completes, semicompletes, and incompletes? (There is also of course the larger question: how typical are Spring Grove ex-patients of American ex-patients in general? We have left it for the most part unanswered.)

**Attrition*

Before we deal with these questions, let us examine some of the most important features of our sample attrition. Like possible sampling bias, attrition held sway at several distinct levels. In Table II-12 is seen the crucial part played in attrition by the sheer amount of recruiting contact which we were able to establish with (1) candidates for the main study who became nonparticipants and (2) candidates for the last-ditch Nonparticipant Study (described below) who once again eluded our data nets. In contact category "None," typically, our recruiting letter was returned undelivered, and it proved impossible either to find the patient in person or to reach him or an effective intermediary by telephone. In the "Minimum" category, the letter apparently went through but elicited no reply; it was subsequently impossible to establish

*Table II-12. Amount of Contact Established with Nonrespondents When Recruiting for Main Study and Nonparticipant Study*

| Contact | Main Study: Nonparticipants | | Nonparticipant Study: Missed Condensed Interview | |
|---|---|---|---|---|
| | *N* | Per Cent | *N* | Per Cent |
| None | 5 | 6 | 7 | 24 |
| Minimum (one-way) | 20 | 25 | 16 | 55 |
| Maximum (two-way) | 54 | 68 | 6 | 21 |
| Total | 79 | ≑100 | 29 | 100 |

further contact by any of our diversified stratagems, including visits to post offices to inquire about forwarding addresses. Only in the "Maximum" category was feedback (always negative, from the subjects in question) actually obtained—by mail, telephone, and/or personal contact.

As Table II-12 indicates, 68 per cent of the 79 recruiting failures in the main study were "persuasion" failures rather than "contact" failures. In the Nonparticipant Study, limited to 79 potential subjects (in contrast to 218 in the main study), contact became the major hurdle: Only 21 per cent of the failures were persuasion failures, while the rate of contact failures ("None" plus "Minimum") jumped to 79 per cent from 31 per cent in the main study.

A second salient question concerning attrition has to do only with those subjects with whom we did succeed in establishing two-way contact. Having been reached, why did they then become non-volunteers? In the last four columns of Table II-13 are shown the answers for the same cases dealt with in Table II-12. Additionally, under "renegers" the same information is tabulated for those patients in the main study who completed Test 1 but who later, by missing Test 12, became classified Incomplete (Figure I-1, boxes E and I; Table I-3). Thus the table above covers *all* attrition except for missed tests Nos. 2 through 11 in the Complete and Semicomplete groups (Figure I-2). To round out the samples, the table's first row includes those cases from whom no reasons were obtained because of incomplete communication. On succeeding rows, the designated reasons emerged from three different recruiting situations. (1) For renegers, the situation was our final but vain effort to schedule monthly testing after Test 1 had been completed but *before* Month 12 had arrived. (2) For nonparticipants (main study), the reason pertained to recruitment for Test 1. (3) In the Nonparticipant Study the reasons were given by those who refused the condensed interview. Note the separate breakdowns for refusals by the patient alone *vs.* otherwise.

"Prohibitive circumstances: impersonal" includes residential moves beyond the study's geographic perimeter, unavailability of suitable informant, and so on. "Unsatisfactory research experience" includes resentment of research staff behavior in our project

*Table II-13. Reasons for Attrition in Main Study and Nonparticipant Study*

| Reason | Main Study: Renegers (Incomplete) | | Main Study: Nonparticipants | | Nonparticipant Study: Missed Condensed Interview | |
|---|---|---|---|---|---|---|
| | *N* | Per Cent | *N* | Per Cent | *N* | Per Cent |
| None: no response to recruiting | | | 25 | 32 | 23 | 79 |
| Unknown: missing data on reason and decider(s) | | | 7 | 9 | | |
| Prohibitive circumstances: impersonal | 10 | 53 | 13 | 16 | | |
| Patient's own decision:[a] | (6) | (32) | (24) | (30) | (6) | (21) |
| Unexplained unwillingness | 2 | 11 | 1 | 1 | | |
| Practical objection | | | 2 | 3 | | |
| Prohibitive circumstances: personal | | | 1 | 1 | 1 | 3 |
| Objection to intrusion | | | 3 | 4 | 1 | 3 |
| Repudiation of patient role | 1 | 5 | 5 | 6 | 1 | 3 |
| Unsatisfactory hospital experience | | | 4 | 5 | | |
| Unsatisfactory research experience | 2 | 11 | 1 | 1 | | |
| Other personal reasons | | | 3 | 4 | 1 | 3 |
| Missing data: reason unknown | 1 | 5 | 4 | 5 | 2 | 7 |
| Patient and/or other person's[b] decision:[a] | (3) | (16) | (10) | (13) | | |
| Unexplained unwillingness | 1 | 5 | 2 | 3 | | |
| Objection to intrusion | 1 | 5 | | | | |
| Repudiation of patient role | | | 1 | 1 | | |
| Unsatisfactory hospital experience | | | 2 | 3 | | |
| Unsatisfactory research experience | 1 | 5 | 1 | 1 | | |
| Other personal reasons | | | 4 | 5 | | |
| Total | 19 | 100 | 79 | 100 | 29 | ≑100 |

[a]Subtotals in parentheses for reasons under this heading.

[b]Most often the nonpatient decision-maker was a potential informant or, less frequently, an informant who had taken one or more earlier tests.

or others, KAS too difficult to understand, and KAS evaluation topics too upsetting. For renegers, the predominating major categories of reasons (Table II-13) were "Prohibitive circumstances: impersonal" and "Patient's own decision"; the majority of nonparticipants were either "no response" or "patient's own decision"; for nonparticipants who missed the condensed interview, there were no notably frequent reasons, as in most instances recruiting did not progress to the point of eliciting any (79 per cent "none: no response to recruiting").

### *Participants Compared with Reference Population*

We now undertake to answer our four questions pertaining to sampling bias. Detailed investigative procedures and results bearing on these questions are given in Appendix N; in the remainder of this chapter, we shall abridge and discuss those findings.

From the Maryland Psychiatric Case Register (Gorwitz, Bahn, Chandler, and Martin, 1963) we were able to obtain various useful statistics on the total Spring Grove ex-patient population. By excluding certain categories of patients (such as organic psychoses) we could estimate with reasonable though not perfect accuracy some of the important characteristics of our sample's reference population. No appreciable discrepancies were observed on four of the five background variables where comparison was possible: age, marital status, education, and diagnosis. On the fifth, our sample did appear to have had more prior hospital admissions than had the Case Register cohort. Sex differences on these variables in the two groups were quite similar, again except on number of hospitalizations prior to last. The heavy female-to-male ratio among participants (Table II-1) was only slightly in excess of the Case Register ratio.

### *Participants Compared with Nonparticipants*

When leaving Spring Grove, participants were decisively more often placed on convalescent leave (as opposed to direct discharge) than were nonparticipants ($p < .001$). We believe that this difference was a key factor in a "separatist" configuration which seems to have characterized nonparticipants and to have been intertwined with their "dropout" status; other findings will be subsumed under this concept. Nonparticipants also tended (not significantly) to be less often married and to have fewer children. Differences were essentially negative on the remaining nine standard background variables.

### **Completes Compared with Nonparticipants: Background and Related Variables*

Expectedly, completes and nonparticipants had roughly the same pattern of background-variable differences and similarities as did participants *vs.* nonparticipants. Of six additional descriptive variables, specially compiled for comparing these two groups, only one–doctor's prognosis when leaving Spring Grove–revealed as much as a borderline difference ($p < .10$): Prognosis tended to be worse for nonparticipants. The two groups were not notably dissimilar as regards type of last admission, clinically rated degree of impairment when released, distance or direction from hospital to home, or monthly rate of accession to the study roster.

### **Completes Compared with Nonparticipants: The Nonparticipant Study*

In many respects, the extent to which completes resembled or differed from nonparticipants is the single most crucial point in the issue of sampling bias; some of our most important data analyses are of necessity based on the complete group alone. Was there a type of patient who had eluded representation in this sample? An adequate answer demanded more information on nonparticipants than had become available in their meager processing in the main study. Accordingly, we designed a special "nonparticipant study" in which, after the posthospital year had ended, a single "Condensed Interview" covering the entire 12 months was conducted with 50 of the nonparticipants.[7] The remaining 29 (37 per cent) proved utterly unreachable. Thus, even in our most definitive effort to specify sampling bias, we were left with an irreduci-

[7]The reduced *N* applies to all remaining results reported on nonparticipants in this chapter, unless otherwise noted. In Appendix N, this group of 50 is termed "nonparticipant-seens."

ble hard core of unresolved opaqueness. Results from the Nonparticipant Study must therefore be read more as suggestive than as conclusive. On the other hand, some of its findings contrasting nonparticipants with completes were so clearly consistent and decisive that they can by no means be disregarded.

Rehospitalization rates during the study year did not significantly discriminate between the 91 completes and 79 nonparticipants, either by number of episodes or number of days in hospital. Forty of the completes (44 per cent) were rehospitalized once or more, as against 30 nonparticipants (38 per cent). Neither was there any clear distinction when nonparticipants were subdivided into those who did and did not undergo the condensed interview.

It proved unfeasible in the nonparticipant study to obtain KAS and stress scores that would have been in any way temporally comparable with those of the completes. The same limitation did not apply to our life situation items, which were by nature less subject to retrospective inaccuracy. It was therefore this set of variables which became the major focus of the condensed interview and the subsequent comparisons of completes with the 50 interviewed nonparticipants.

Four of the main study's life situation areas were covered, with a total of 46 tests for differences: home and family (14 tests); work and homemaking (12 tests); outpatient treatment (13 tests); and drug treatment (7 tests). Throughout the first two areas, no convincing differences were found, except that female homemakers in the "complete" group functioned more responsibly, especially at Month 1. It was in the areas of outpatient and drug treatment that the most decisive indications of probable sampling bias became manifest.

Completes were found to have been much more involved in aftercare treatment than nonparticipants throughout the posthospital year—especially as regarded the Spring Grove Outpatient Clinic. The same contrast held for treatment by nonpsychiatric physicians, but with an interesting paradoxical exception: Considering only the anchor months 1 and 12, we found that it was the nonparticipants, not the completes, who visited physicians significantly more often at these particular periods.

In the Nonparticipant-Study investigation of drug treatment we emphasized actual consumption of medication. In this area, completes exceeded nonparticipants even more decisively than in outpatient treatment—not only as to the proportion who took at least some drug during the year (96 per cent *vs.* 66 per cent), but also on more specific indexes of the actual amount of medicine taken.

Inasmuch as completes were much more often on convalescent leave from Spring Grove than were nonparticipants, it is conceivable that this background variable may in itself have predetermined the preponderance of completes in aftercare treatment: hospital policy is slanted accordingly. However, results of special analyses, with type of release controlled, did not confirm this hypothesis. On a clear majority of the variables tested, the observed treatment differences persisted despite the type-of-release control.

In one other test for deceptive effects in our results, we treated as an independent variable the amount of time elapsed between the end of the nonparticipant's posthospital year and his condensed interview—a variable with considerable unavoidable range from minimum to maximum. Time-lag effects did appear in the interview reports. However, directional trends indicated that, had these effects *not* been present, the observed differences between completes and nonparticipants might have been *greater* rather than smaller. Furthermore, lag effect seemed to have functioned primarily where interview items pertained to Month 1 or called for highly specific information.

Is it possible to synthesize and interpret all of these results so as to postulate any pattern of clinical or motivational attributes by which nonparticipants might be characterized as meaningfully different from completes? We can now propose an affirmative hypothesis. Six strands of evidence converge persuasively to support the separatism configuration first noted in conjunction with type-of-release differences. (1) All nonparticipants were individuals who, by definition, had eluded concerted efforts to enlist them in a research project affiliated with the hospital where they once had been inpatients. (2) Nonparticipants were more often discharged outright from Spring Grove, as opposed to being placed on convalescent leave, than were their "complete" counterparts (28 per cent *vs.* 12 per cent, $p < .02$). Quite often, at Spring Grove, the departing patient or his family, or both, participate actively with the doctor in the choice of convalescent leave or discharge. If (as the evidence suggests) the entire group of nonparticipants left the hospital with a somewhat poorer average clinical prognosis and impairment rating than completes, then there may have had to be more than usual pressure from patient and relatives for outright discharge, since clinical policy for these patients would ordinarily have been slanted toward convalescent leave as a safeguard. (3) Although the difference was not significant, nonparticipants as a whole were more often single, divorced, separated, or widowed, while completes were more often married. (4) Nonparticipant female homemakers showed less domestic responsibility than completes. (5) On several counts, nonparticipants were less involved in outpatient aftercare during the posthospital study year. The one notable exception was that, at Months 1 and 12 considered jointly, nonparticipants significantly exceeded completes in frequency of visits to nonpsychiatric physicians (probably family doctors in most instances). Here, even while treatment was sought, affiliation with Spring Grove via its Outpatient Clinic was avoided. (6) Nonparticipants were likewise much more sparing than completes in using medication, a token par excellence of clinical involvement and continuing identity as a psychiatric patient. In a study of ex-patients' consumption of prescribed aftercare drugs, Nickerson, Epps, and Heckel (1966) concluded: "In general, drug avoiders are highly mobile and unstable in their residence, marriage, employment history, and other social behaviors such as church attendance, while those following prescribed drug therapy are more settled and conforming."

While nonconformity may well have been generalized as a style of life in many of our nonparticipants, in the present context it can be understood more specifically—and more confidently—as a defense employed in coping with the fact of having been a mental hospital patient. One suspects that the clinically familiar phenomenon of denial of illness was indigenous to the separatist configuration (Hankoff, Engelhardt, Freedman, Mann, and Margolis, 1960).

Among some of our participants who cooperated minimally and reluctantly with our research requirements, there was a tendency to endorse the following two statements (plus a few others) as retrospective explanations of their elusiveness: "I did not want to have any more contact with Spring Grove," and "I did not want to think about mental illness." A few of these individuals quite literally denied illness in their own voluntary comments. One wrote: "I did not feel mentally upset, just a physical invalid. . . . In the first place I was sent to Spring Grove because of a painful condition in my mouth, not mentally upset. All very disgusting." Another complained: "There seems to be too much concernment in my case. . . . They found nothing wrong with me when I got there" (Michaux, Michaux, Esser, and Oliver, 1968). Among nonparticipants, a similarly scornful outlook seemed to pervade the "condensed interview" climate when, as often happened, the interviewer found them brusque and distant. In contrast, the research staff had earlier noticed and discussed the characteristically obliging, loyal, and emotionally dependent attitudes of those patients who faithfully kept most or all of their test appointments in the main study. Thus we came to feel that, however sick any nonparticipants were, those who refused Test 1 may have been striving more actively toward health than those participants who seemed to experience testing as one answer to their need to maintain ties with the hospital, staking their security on continuing their roles as patients.

### *Differences among Completes, Semicompletes, and Incompletes

Comparisons among these three data groups are also of relevance to the issue of sampling bias, inasmuch as completes are included in all major data analyses, semicompletes of necessity only in some, and incompletes in still fewer. As will be seen in the next chapter (Tables III-1, III-2, III-3, and III-4), rehospitalization throughout the posthospital year was disproportionately excessive in the complete group—significantly so, when tested parametrically—while semicompletes differed little from incompletes. When the three groups were compared at each of the 12 months separately (Appendix N, Table N-8), completes often showed decisively more frequent rehospitalization than semicompletes or incompletes, whose rates were again similar to each other's. This pattern of differences tended to concentrate within Months 4 through 9 and was not marked at Month 1 or 12.

None of the differences on the twelve background variables reached the .05 significance level and only one was borderline ($p < .10$): type of release, with completes having the highest proportion of patients on convalescent leave (88 per cent) and with semicompletes and incompletes having almost identical proportions. Thus, within the participant sample, the association between type of release and research accessibility is in the same direction as in the comparison of completes with nonparticipants.

Each of the 26 adjustment variables and the 40 life situation variables was tested for data-group differences at Month 1. The same analyses were made at Month 12, but were here limited necessarily to completes *vs.* semicompletes. At both months the paucity of significant discriminations appeared well within random expectations. On the adjustment variables in particular, if one assumes that any real differences had existed, ample and decisive statistical indications of such differences would have been expected in view of the often high intercorrelations among these measures (Appendix M, Table M-1). Differences in "adjustment" and "life situation" were not tested at Months 2 and 11; from the evidence available there is little or no ground for suspecting sampling bias at these points.

## *Implications of Sampling Bias for the Study's Findings*

There can be little doubt that, had there been no attrition among our 218 eligible selectees, the study sample would have been by operational definition random and presumptively representative. But we must now take into account the discernible sampling bias which did develop in conjunction with considerable attrition.

Available evidence, though somewhat meager, indicates that participants probably did not differ drastically from the reference population of Spring Grove ex-patients. Nor is there proof that participants, or complete cases only, differed from nonparticipants in any terms specifiable *while they were still inpatients.* It was only when our candidates had reached the hospital door, en routc back to the community, that the first cogent sign of sampling bias in the form of "type of release" was revealed.

By contriving to learn as much as possible about our nonparticipants' posthospital year, we have established rather conclusively that they participated comparatively little in aftercare, including but not limited to medication. In contextual perspective, this behavior identifies them psychodynamically as persons intent on maintaining defensive distance from the hospital and from its outpatient arm (as well as from our hospital-affiliated research project). Provocative though this proposition may be, it throws but little light on the issue of sampling bias. If pursued, it can only raise the question: In what way would our findings have been different, if these separatists had been included in our data? But the question is academic, for, if nonparticipants had been constitutionally includable, they could not constitutionally have been separatists!

The weight of the sampling-bias evidence, and of its implications for our results, must hence inhere mainly in the purely empirical differences between completes and nonparticipants as regards type of release and participation in aftercare. Thus the decisive question is: How different would our obtained results have been in a sample more fairly representative by virtue of containing larger proportions of (1) patients directly discharged from Spring Grove and (2) patients involved little or none in aftercare?

Our answer is based on a forward look at results to be presented, momentarily considering these two conditions as control variables and assuming negligible interaction effects differentially influencing complete and nonparticipant data. From this viewpoint, a less biased study sample should have (1) attained on the average *better* adjustment scores—both at anchor Months 1 and 12 as well as longitudinally throughout the posthospital year, and (2) contained somewhat *fewer* relapsers. The two major sampling-bias conditions agree in these indications. We shall leave it largely to the reader to mentally tag them and to trace their qualifying ramifications throughout our reported results.[8]

## SUMMARY

Eight rules of thumb are stated, generally applicable to analysis and presentation of results throughout the study. Attention to them is essential for reader orientation.

The 139 participants averaged 41.1 years of age and had a mean education of 10.4 years. Characteristically but not exclusively, they were Protestant (61.2 per cent) females (68.3 per cent), married, with children, and with little or no pre-study work history.

As regards hospitalization and illness, the distribution spectrums were broad. About three-fourths of the sample had had more than one psychiatric hospitalization. The median length of the last or only hospitalization was 2.4 months. Most participants were psychotic (74.8 per cent), predominately schizophrenic (54.7 per cent).

Descriptive findings on early posthospital adjustment and life situation are based on the first of twelve monthly evaluations directly following release from the hospital and recruitment for the study. At Month 1, the participants were evidently somewhat sicker than normals, but considerably less sick than day center patients and about-to-be-hospitalized inpatients as revealed by

[8]It may seem surprising and paradoxical that by adding *less*-treated patients to our sample we would have improved adjustment scores and decreased rehospitalization rates; it will not seem so after perusal of later findings. It is true that, in terms of prognosis and impairment at time of release, nonparticipants seemed sicker than completes, insofar as clinical data were available (Appendix N, Table N-3). However, quite a few cases are missing from both groups in these analyses; they reflect the clinical judgment of various psychiatrists; and none of our other findings agree with the prognosis and impairment comparison. Aside from statistical inferences, we have already noted the possible healthiness of the act of refusing to participate in our research, as well as the possible pathological dependency implicit in regular participation. Discussions with the chief of the Spring Grove Outpatient Clinic disclosed that similar dependency was observable in many of its aftercare patients, who often had to be "weaned" from clinic attendance. Thus our completes were quite likely motivated by needs almost the converse of our nonparticipants' separatism. We further believe that, for the completes, aftercare surveillance militated in favor of higher rehospitalization rates—not only by way of sheer clinical monitoring, making it increasingly likely that readmission would be proposed, but also by way of patient psychodynamics, entailing greater willingness to accept readmission once it was proposed.

KAS comparisons involving other Maryland studies. The 26 adjustment variables exhibited numerous high intercorrelations, but were negligibly correlated with five key background variables. Among the five key background variables themselves, four out of ten correlations were significant and three of the four involved sex. Sex was also significantly related to some of the other background variables.

Life-situation interviews covering Month 1 indicated that domestic relations were typically with spouse and children; parents figured less frequently. Gainful employment was unusual, but females were carrying considerable responsibility as homemakers. Four patients in five were receiving aftercare; the prime facility was the Spring Grove Outpatient Clinic and the prime treatment was chemotherapy. A noteworthy amount of environmental stress was reported on the Stress Inquiry, a specially designed provisional interview technique used for the first time in the present study.

To check on the generality of all findings, considerable investigative effort was devoted to the question of sampling bias. It was concluded that, had the sample been more precisely representative, monthly adjustment scores would probably have been somewhat better and the proportion of relapsers somewhat smaller. Psychodynamically, nonparticipants appeared to be separatists—in reference not only to the project but also to inpatient and aftercare treatment.

Chapter III

# Course of Adjustment

In our conceptual framework, the term "course of adjustment" held a commanding position. By dividing the posthospital year into twelve monthly evaluation segments, we aimed to depict more precisely, and hopefully to understand more effectively, some of the salient conditions and processes working for and against the patient during this critical period. Accordingly it is this chapter which, as compared with other follow-up studies, contains our most distinctive findings, i.e., those stemming most directly from the longitudinal repeated-measurements procedure. Essential to our approach has been maximum use of prospective as opposed to retrospective formulations, both here and in subsequent chapters. We hope that such an approach can point the way toward more effective operational models for outpatient clinical practice—including, but not necessarily limited to, aftercare. We are particularly mindful of clinicians' needs to be able to identify, before it is too late, the patient for whom hospitalization is becoming an imminent danger—and also the patient who, with or without such a danger, may need a change in the individualized planning of his ongoing outpatient treatment.

## REHOSPITALIZATION

By any psychometric standards, hospitalization *vs.* non-hospitalization within a given time span is at best a crude and untrustworthy index of in-community adjustment. When used as an estimate of psychiatric morbidity in whatever context, its limitations are similar to those of the death rate in public health statistics. Concerning the latter, the Director of the National Center for Health Statistics has remarked: "The death rate, and indeed the entire battery of vital statistics that have long been collected by the states and the Federal Government, no longer yield enough information on which to base a sound national health policy" (Linder, 1966).

From the clinician's standpoint, however, hospitalization is a matter of cardinal importance—whether viewed prospectively as a therapeutic decision or retrospectively as an episode in the patient's unfolding history. Prevention of hospitalization is currently the target of enormous professional effort. Community mental health programs are now vigorously emphasizing constructive alternatives to inpatient treatment. But the data-collection period in our project was for the most part too early for our patients to benefit from these emerging alternatives. Thus, in studying their course of posthospital adjustment, we must deal with rehospitalization as a major fact of life—an abrupt interruption of the patient's effort to attain stable in-community living, and an event which perforce occasioned many gaps in our longitudinal evaluations of that adjustment.

Among Maryland residents, recent trends toward more frequent admissions and discharges seem to have neither aggravated nor mitigated the problem of rehospitalization. In February, 1963, when our first subjects were being recruited, the state-wide situation was described as follows in a bulletin from the Department of Mental Hygiene:

> Has the rapid decline in the average length of hospitalization produced a proportionally greater number of former patients who are not capable of adjusting to the environment outside the hospital confines? Available data indicate that this is not correct. . . . From . . . 1954 to . . . 1962 . . . the annual ratio of one readmission for every two discharges has remained almost constant. . . . The ratio of readmissions to the number of Maryland residents who have ever been hospitalized for a psychiatric illness is not believed to have changed greatly in recent years and may actually have declined. . . . Because of the anticipated continuing increase in discharges, the

number of readmissions can be expected to increase also. (Tuerk and Gorwitz, 1963a.)

An overview of our patients' readmission experience during the study year is shown in Figure III-1. Only the first readmission (out of a maximum of three) was counted in plotting the three participant lines. Their noncumulative readmission line indicates no pronounced monthly "zones" of danger or safety, though the greatest frequency was at Month 2 and the smallest at Month 3. The cumulative participant line shows that 21.6 per cent of the 139 participants had been rehospitalized by Month 6; at the end of the year the overall rate had reached 37.4 per cent.[1]

Within each of the three data-groups, most patients remained unrehospitalized for the entire year (Table III-1). One or more rehospitalizations occurred for 44 per cent of the completes but only for 24 per cent of the semicompletes and 26 per cent of incompletes. Frequency of readmission thus tends to be associated with frequency of completing the research tests. We have already postulated that the stronger emotional affiliation with treatment facilities, attributed to completes, may have generalized to induce greater research participation. From another standpoint, their frequent KAS testing may well have induced keener self-consciousness concerning their symptoms, which in turn may have made them more likely to initiate or accept rehospitalization.

[1]Several points should be made about the participants' rehospitalization rates, especially as compared cumulatively with the Maryland Case Register findings. (1) The Case Register's Spring Grove cohort was quite similar to ours in terms of diagnosis and of operational definition of hospital release and readmission; its follow-up period overlapped our own in calendar time. (2) The Case Register cohort differed from our participants in three noteworthy aspects: it covered a total population as defined with no attrition; age was limited to a minimum of 25 and a maximum of 54; and the maximum length of most rehospitalizations was set at one year. (3) If the participant sample had included the three patients who had become ineligible by relapsing during the first 20 posthospital days, the Month-1 percentage would read 5.0 instead of 2.9, and subsequent monthly cumulative percentages would be correspondingly higher. (4) For the small group of 19 incompletes, our rehospitalization rates may have been underestimated: Coverage of their possible admission to hospitals other than Spring Grove was at best sporadic, and they were of course not interrogated at Month 12. Inasmuch as their rate of admission to other hospitals may have been as high as 11 per cent (Gorwitz, Bahn, Klee, and Solomon, 1966, p. 1102), we may have overlooked about 2 of the incomplete cases' rehospitalizations (1.4 per cent of all participants). (5) On the other hand, we have already established from the investigation of sampling bias that the project's attrition could have spuriously *increased* our obtained rehospitalization rates.

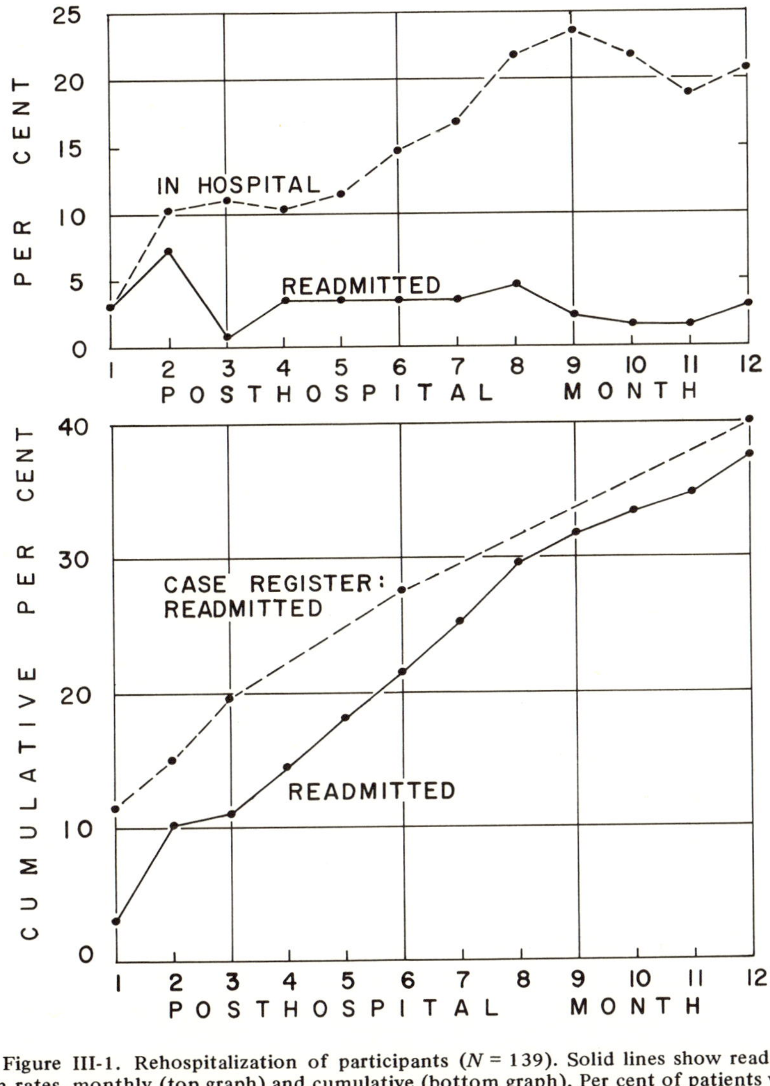


Figure III-1. Rehospitalization of participants ($N = 139$). Solid lines show readmission rates, monthly (top graph) and cumulative (bottom graph). Per cent of patients who were confined to hospital at each month is shown by broken line in top graph. In bottom graph, broken line is based on a reasonably comparable, larger cohort of 775 Spring Grove patients whose rehospitalizations were tabulated by the Maryland Psychiatric Case Register (U.S. Department of Health, Education and Welfare, and Maryland Department of Mental Hygiene, 1966, Vol. 1, p. 6).

Most patients who did re-enter the hospital accumulated at least two months of inpatient time during the year, with a maximum of

*Table III-1. Number of Rehospitalizations*

| Number of Rehospitalizations | Complete | | Semicomplete | | Incomplete | | Total | |
|---|---|---|---|---|---|---|---|---|
| | *N* | Per Cent | *N* | Per Cent | *N* | Per Cent | *N* | Per Cent |
| None | 51 | 56 | 22 | 76 | 14 | 74 | 87 | 62.6 |
| One | 33 | 36 | 5 | 17 | 5 | 26 | 43 | 30.9 |
| Two or three[a] | 7 | 8 | 2 | 7 | 0 | 0 | 9 | 6.5 |
| Total | 91 | 100 | 29 | 100 | 19 | 100 | 139 | 100.0 |

$\chi^2 = 5.98, p < .25$

[a]Only one patient, a male in the "complete" group, was rehospitalized three times.

11 months (Table III-2). In terms of inpatient days, completes again outranked the other two groups who differed little from each other. The completes' average of 59.0 inpatient days was significantly greater than the average for semicompletes pooled

*Table III-2. Total Days Rehospitalized: Gross Distributions*

| Number of Days | Complete | | Semicomplete | | Incomplete | | Total | |
|---|---|---|---|---|---|---|---|---|
| | *N* | Per Cent | *N* | Per Cent | *N* | Per Cent | *N* | Per Cent |
| None | 51 | 56 | 22 | 76 | 14 | 74 | 87 | 62.6 |
| 1 to 59 | 10 | 11 | 2 | 7 | 2 | 11 | 14 | 10.1 |
| 60 to 321 | 30 | 33 | 5 | 17 | 3 | 16 | 38 | 27.3 |
| Total | 91 | 100 | 29 | 100 | 19 | ÷100 | 139 | 100.0 |

$\chi^2 = 5.25, p < .30$

with incompletes (Table III-3, $t = 2.59, p < .02$). The difference becomes more pronounced when we consider only the relapsers, i.e., those patients who had at least one rehospitalization during

*Table III-3. Total Days Rehospitalized: Means, Standard Deviations, and Ranges*

| Statistic | Complete | Semicomplete | Incomplete | All Participants |
|---|---|---|---|---|
| *N* | 91 | 29 | 19 | 139 |
| Mean | 59.0 | 21.9 | 25.2 | 46.6 |
| S. D. | 88.5 | 46.5 | 51.2 | 78.9 |
| Range | 0 to 321 | 0 to 188 | 0 to 188 | 0 to 321 |

the year (Table III-4, $t = 15.44$, $p < .001$). As Tables III-3 and III-4 indicate, the entire sample of participants averaged 46.6 days rehospitalized and the 52 relapsers averaged 124.7 days.

*Table III-4. Total Days Rehospitalized: Medians, Means, Standard Deviations, and Ranges (Relapsers Only)*

| Statistic | Complete | Semicomplete | Incomplete | All Relapsers |
|---|---|---|---|---|
| *N* | 40 | 7 | 5 | 52 |
| Median | 126.0 | 79.0 | 67.0 | 113.5 |
| Mean | 134.3 | 90.7 | 95.6 | 124.7 |
| S. D. | 87.8 | 52.2 | 56.8 | 83.2 |
| Range | 1 to 321 | 29 to 188 | 34 to 188 | 1 to 321 |

## TREATMENT AT MONTH 1: SOME SPECIAL QUESTIONS

In a sense, the Month-1 treatment situation is a pivotal factor in the patient's return from hospital to community. Hence the question naturally arises: Who were the 19 participants who by their own report had no drug prescribed whatever during Month 1 (Table II-8)? One would have expected them to be predominately nonpsychotic, more often on direct discharge from Spring Grove, and comparatively well-adjusted; these are the familiar guidelines for chemotherapeutic decisions. When the 19 drug-free patients were compared with the remaining 120 participants, expectations were decisively confirmed as regards diagnosis and type of release, as indicated in Table III-5. These two background variables proved highly interrelated ($p < .005$): 37 per cent of all nonpsychotic participants were out on direct discharge, as against 9 per cent of the schizophrenics and 14 per cent of the patients with other psychoses. To test the expected relationship between adjustment and drug prescription, we had recourse to a KAS global adjustment score—here used for the first time in our analyses and statistically defined in Appendix O. As Table III-5 indicates, there was only a slight tendency for drug-free patients to score better than the median for all participants on this composite measure. It should be noted, however, that virtually all of the drug-

*Table III-5. Patients with No Drug Prescribed at Month 1 (N = 19): Distributions by Diagnosis, Type of Release, and Month-1 Global Adjustment*

| Item | *N* | Per Cent[a] |
|---|---|---|
| Diagnosis ($p < .005$): | | |
| Schizophrenic reaction | 6 | 8 |
| Psychoses other than schizophrenia | 2 | 7 |
| Nonpsychotic disorders | 11 | 31 |
| Type of release ($p < .001$): | | |
| Convalescent leave | 9 | 7.8 |
| Discharge | 10 | 42 |
| Month-1 global adjustment ($p < .25$): | | |
| Worse than median | 7 | 10 |
| Better than median | 12 | 17 |

[a]Of all schizophrenic reactions, all psychoses other than schizophrenia, and so on.

prescription decisions were made considerably earlier than the end of Month 1, on which the global adjustment scores are based.

Viewed in a different perspective, the Month-1 treatment situation was one of the points of departure for a 12-month observation period. It may have changed later; how was its monthly course related to course of adjustment? Many specific questions are implied by this general one. For the moment, let us consider only the 52 relapsers. Did they begin the year with, or without, treatment? Equally or more important—what was their treatment situation during the critical period immediately preceding their first or only rehospitalization? Figure III-2 deals with these questions in regard to the 49 relapsers for whom all relevant data were available. Of these 49 patients, 82 per cent were in outpatient treatment at Month 1 and 76 per cent used a drug at that time. As for the pre-relapse period, we find by summing adjacent light-shaded percentages that, again, 82 per cent were in outpatient treatment (though they were not all the same identical individuals), while the percentage using drug had dropped to 57. Examining the original data more closely, we ascertained that 40 of the 49 relapsers were in outpatient treatment at Month 1, and 36 of the same 40 (90 per cent) were still in treatment at the pre-relapse period; similarly, 37 relapsers (76 per cent) were using drug at Month 1, but only 22 of them (59 per cent) were still using it at

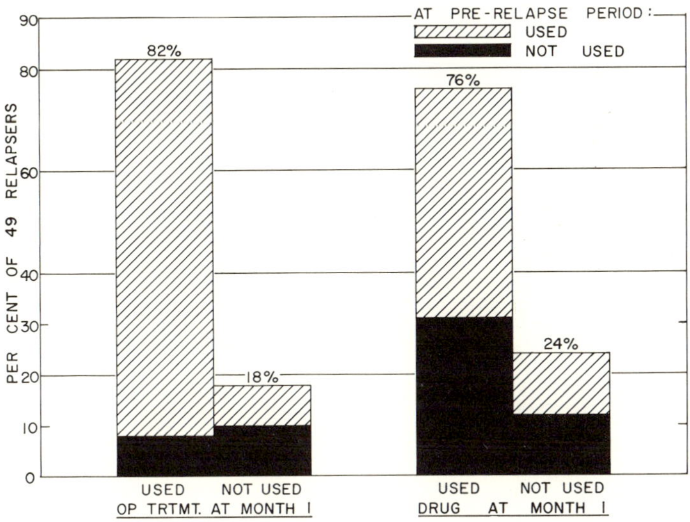


**Figure III-2.** Use of outpatient treatment and drug, at Month 1 and at first or only pre-relapse period, by 49 relapsers. Based on patient's report in life-situation interview. For the total of 52 relapsers, data are missing on three who failed to take the relapse test.

the pre-relapse period. (A few other cases, of course, were negative at Month 1 and positive at pre-relapse; still others were negative at both periods.) For all 49 relapsers, we find that continued participation in outpatient treatment at pre-relapse is predictable from participation at Month 1 ($\chi^2 = 7.36$, $p < .01$). But a similar forecast from Month 1 is not possible for pre-relapse drug usage ($\chi^2 = 0.33$, $p < .70$).[2] Further inspection of raw data indicated that the decline in drug usage at pre-relapse was due almost entirely to fewer prescriptions, not to patients' failure to use prescribed drugs. (At Month 1, all patients who had a drug prescribed were using it; at pre-relapse, there were only two patients who were failing to use a prescribed drug.) Could some of these relapses have been prevented by more drug prescriptions? Probably so, according to other research evidence (Engelhardt, Freedman, Glick, Hankoff, Mann, and Margolis, 1960; Gross, Hitchman, Reeves, Lawrence, and Newell, 1961)–though there are investi-

[2]Based on four-cell contingency tables, partitioned in the same manner as by columns and shading in Figure III-2.

gators who doubtless would hesitate to agree (Hughes and Little, 1967; Reilly, Wilson, and McClinton, 1967).

## NONRELAPSERS COMPARED WITH RELAPSERS

### *Adjustment*

Throughout the posthospital year, monthly differences in adjustment between nonrelapsers and relapsers were strikingly manifold and sizable. Comparisons were made by *t* tests at each month, on each of the 26 adjustment variables. Of the 312 tests thus made, 143 (nearly half) were significant at or beyond the .05 level, and nonrelapsers invariably had the significantly better mean adjustment score.

These comparisons, summarized in Table III-6, were subject to several special conditions. Only the 91 complete cases (51 nonrelapsers, 40 relapsers) could be used, because of the need for longitudinal sample consistency. Even so, *N*s fluctuated from month to month because of the few tests illegitimately missed (Figure I-2) plus the many tests legitimately missed by relapsers when they were rehospitalized. Most importantly, this particular compilation of data is by no means methodologically "clean:" at any typical single month, relapsers who have not yet been rehospitalized are commingled with other relapsers who are back in the community after having been readmitted and released. Hence it would be improper to interpret this analysis either prospectively or retrospectively; it is better viewed simply as a series of 12 monthly cross-sections. (Even at Month 1, results should not be thought of in terms of predicting later relapse, for at that period there were already two patients who were back in hospital, and who took a relapse test for Month 1.) What we are dealing with in this analysis is, in effect, monthly differences in in-community adjustment between those patients who did and those who did not undergo rehospitalization, with or without subsequent release, during the posthospital year.

The results as a whole, reflecting as they do overwhelmingly better adjustment on the part of nonrelapsers, indicate that those patients who underwent rehospitalization were indeed those who needed it most. Except for Month 2, significant differences occurred most densely toward the end of the year (Months 9, 11, 12) and least densely toward the beginning (Months 1, 3, 4)—a trend that is not easily interpretable, though it does suggest that rehospitalization did not improve adjustment, inasmuch as patients who had been readmitted and subsequently released were obviously more numerous at later months.

Reading down the first column in Table III-6, we find that the four variables which discriminated most often from month to month were *Sus* (Suspiciousness), *Biz* (Bizarreness), *SEA-I* (Performance of Socially-Expected Activities–Informant), and *FTA-I* (Free-Time Activities–Informant). Closely following, in order of frequency of monthly discrimination, were *Anx* (Anxiety), *Psy* (General Psychopathology), *Sta* (Emotional Stability), and *SFA-I* (Satisfaction with Free-Time Activities–Informant). Three of the KAS patient self-report scales showed no significant difference between nonrelapsers and relapsers at any single month and are hence not shown in Table III-6: *Sym* (Symptom Discomfort), *SSA-P* (Satisfaction with Socially-Expected Activities–Patient), *FTA-P* (Free-Time Activities–Patient). Likewise, the two stress variables were largely negative for differences: *Str-P* (Patient Stress), with none significant at any month (hence not included in table) and *Str-I* (Informant Stress), discriminating only at Month 11. When designing the project, we had expected the two stress indexes to show relatively high scores antecedently associated with rehospitalization, since environmental stress is often blamed for admissions. In this instance, however, their failure to discriminate between nonrelapsers and relapsers could be related to the methodological impurities of these data, as noted above.

Table III-6 represents the first of several analyses in which critical questions of posthospital adjustment are dealt with by testing all 26 adjustment variables across the board. When one considers the results of such analyses, a question of intrinsic interest has to do with the source of the information, i.e., patient *vs.* informant. Among whatever significant results are obtained, is one of the two respondents represented more heavily than the other? Pursuit of this question should serve not only to illuminate psychosocial processes in our own study, but also to provide guidelines for choosing respondents when designing further research studies and

*Table III-6. Significant Monthly Differences in Adjustment between Nonrelapsers and Relapsers (Complete Cases Only)*

| Variable | No. of Mos. Sig. | Significant Results: By Month No.: *p* 1 | 2 | 3 | 4 | 5 | 6 | 7 | 8 | 9 | 10 | 11 | 12 |
|---|---|---|---|---|---|---|---|---|---|---|---|---|---|
| KAS–Patient (see also Informant below): | | | | | | | | | | | | | |
| *SEA-P* | 8 | .01 | .01 | .01 | .05 | .001 | .05 | * | * | .05 | * | * | .05 |
| *LOE-P* | 3 | * | * | .05 | * | .05 | * | .05 | * | * | * | * | * |
| *SFA-P* | 6 | .05 | * | * | .05 | .05 | .02 | * | * | * | * | .01 | .05 |
| KAS–Informant only: | | | | | | | | | | | | | |
| *Bel* | 6 | * | * | * | * | * | * | .01 | .001 | .01 | .02 | .02 | .05 |
| *Exp* | 1 | * | * | * | * | * | * | * | * | * | * | .05 | * |
| *Neg* | 6 | * | .01 | * | * | * | * | * | .01 | .01 | .05 | .05 | .01 |
| *Hel* | 6 | * | .01 | * | * | * | .02 | .02 | * | .01 | * | .05 | .01 |
| *Sus* | 10 | .05 | .05 | * | * | .05 | .01 | .01 | .01 | .01 | .05 | .01 | .05 |
| *Anx* | 9 | * | .001 | * | * | .05 | .001 | .001 | .02 | .001 | .05 | .01 | .001 |
| *Wdl* | 2 | .02 | .05 | * | * | * | * | * | * | * | * | * | * |
| *Psy* | 9 | .01 | .001 | * | * | * | .01 | .001 | .01 | .001 | .05 | .01 | .02 |
| *Ner* | 7 | * | .02 | * | .05 | .05 | * | .02 | * | .01 | * | .01 | .01 |
| *Con* | 5 | * | .02 | .02 | * | * | .05 | * | * | .02 | * | .01 | * |
| *Biz* | 10 | * | .01 | * | .05 | .02 | .01 | .001 | .01 | .001 | .05 | .01 | .02 |
| *Hyp* | 7 | * | .001 | * | * | * | .01 | .001 | .01 | .01 | * | .01 | .01 |
| *Sta* | 9 | .02 | .01 | * | .02 | .05 | * | * | .01 | .01 | .02 | .01 | .02 |

| | | | | | | | | | | | | | |
|---|---|---|---|---|---|---|---|---|---|---|---|---|---|
| KAS–Informant (see also Patient above): | | | | | | | | | | | | | |
| *SEA-I* | 10 | .02 | .01 | .05 | .01 | .05 | * | * | .02 | .01 | .01 | .01 | .001 |
| *LOE-I* | 2 | * | * | * | * | * | * | * | * | * | .02 | .05 | * |
| *SSA-I* | 5 | * | .05 | * | .05 | * | .02 | * | * | .01 | .05 | * | * |
| *FTA-I* | 12 | .001 | .001 | .001 | .01 | .01 | .001 | .01 | .01 | .001 | .01 | .01 | .001 |
| *SFA-I* | 9 | .02 | .01 | .05 | .05 | * | .02 | .05 | * | .01 | * | .05 | .01 |
| Stress Index: | | | | | | | | | | | | | |
| *Str-I* | 1 | * | * | * | * | * | * | * | * | * | * | .05 | * |
| Nonrelapsers: *N* | | 51 | 49 | 48 | 45 | 49 | 49 | 50 | 49 | 51 | 50 | 47 | 51 |
| Relapsers: *N* | | 40 | 37 | 21 | 27 | 24 | 23 | 22 | 18 | 16 | 19 | 21 | 21 |

*Nonrelapsers and relapsers not significantly different.

when using the KAS clinically with individual treatment cases. Seven of the 26 adjustment variables are based on the patient's self-report; the remaining 19 utilize the informant as a lay observer reporting on the patient (Table II-3). By simple tabulations and percentage calculations, it is easy to tell whether in a given analysis either respondent is contributing more than his expected share of significant results. In the case of Table III-6, the informant clearly outdistanced the patient in this respect—whether the tally is based on all 312 *t* tests, or simply on which of the 26 adjustment variables discriminated significantly during at least one month. The informant's "superiority" in this context may stem from any of three conditions, and we suspect that all three are involved: (1) The informant's observing and reporting, largely unclouded by any mental illness of his own, are actually more valid than the patient's. (2) In transactions having to do with the patient's remaining at home *vs.* returning to the hospital, close relatives of the patient (such as those who served as our informants) often function as powerful arbiters. (3) As the year progressed, and some of the relapsers returned home and resumed testing, the sheer fact of their rehospitalization could have predisposed informants to perceive them as sicker than those patients who had succeeded in remaining out of the hospital—quite apart from the actual severity of existing illness.

Disregarding the respondent's identity, we may also consider the 26 adjustment variables in terms of their manifest content. Sixteen of them are classifiable as psychopathological, four as social, and six as judgmental. (See Appendix P for rationale and listing of these groupings.) We shall use this schema, as well as the patient-informant dichotomy, as a framework for examining findings on adjustment variables. When it is applied to Table III-6, it shows no real difference among the three categories as regards variables yielding at least one significant monthly discrimination; however, when each monthly *t* test is counted separately, comparatively heavy weight is carried by the social variables, while the psychopathological variables carry exactly their expected share and the judgmental variables are somewhat underrepresented.

We may think of nonrelapsers and relapsers as two contrasting "treatment groups": the latter received inpatient treatment during the posthospital year, while the former did not. (Both groups received some outpatient treatment; as will be shown, relapsers may have surpassed nonrelapsers in this respect.) By the same token, in-community adjustment as measured at Month 12 can be viewed as a "post-treatment" evaluation—bearing in mind that for such an evaluation we must redefine our sample. Complete and semi-complete cases can be included, but not incompletes. From the 120 cases thus available we must subtract 22 relapsers who were back in the hospital throughout Month 12 and therefore took no test at that time; we cannot say how, or to what extent, their exclusion affects the nonrelapser-relapser comparison.[3] Additionally, we have excluded from this and all similar end-of-year analyses four relapser cases who completed a *relapse* test at Month 12: since these patients spent part of Month 12 in the community and the remainder in the hospital, their sample-membership status for Month-12 analyses was considered equivocal. Thus the total $N$ of 120 for analyses of this kind is reduced to 94 (73 nonrelapsers plus 21 relapsers). We shall refer to this group as the anchor-months cohort.

For the "post-treatment" comparison, each of the 26 adjustment variables was subjected to analysis of covariance, holding constant the Month-1 score on the same variable so as to take into account initial differences. One cannot confidently forecast the outcome of such tests. By virtue of having received more drastic treatment, relapsers could conceivably be less sick than nonrelapsers at Month 12; or, having been sicker all along throughout the year, relapsers might remain so at Month 12; or finally, these two contrasting processes might cancel each other out, leaving essentially no differences between the two groups.

The covariance analysis yielded unambiguous results on 5 of the 26 adjustment variables: see Table III-7, which shows relapsers to have been consistently sicker than nonrelapsers at Month 12, when allowance is made for reversed score directions on *SEA-I* and *LOE-I* (Level of Expectations–Informant). On the remaining 21

[3]We do know by $t$ tests that those relapsers who at Month 12 were *in* the hospital did not differ significantly from those who were *out*, on age ($p < .20$), education ($p < .60$), years hospitalized prior to last admission ($p < .90$), or months hospitalized during last admission ($p < .30$).

*Table III-7. Adjustment Variables Showing Greatest Differences between 73 Nonrelapsers and 21 Relapsers at Month 12*

| Variable | Adjusted Mean at Month 12 | | Covariance Results | |
|---|---|---|---|---|
| | Nonrelapsers | Relapsers | *F* | *p* |
| *SSA-P* | 6.4 | 12.3 | 7.89 | .01 |
| *SFA-P* | 27.7 | 30.5 | 4.17 | .05 |
| *Anx (I)* | 6.6 | 7.7 | 5.58 | .025 |
| *SEA-I* | 35.9 | 33.8 | 3.09 | .10 |
| *LOE-I* | 37.6 | 35.5 | 3.48 | .10 |

variables, discriminations were vitiated by nonsignificant covariance *F*s and/or significant regression *F*s. Nonetheless, adjusted Month-12 means showed relapsers to be sicker than nonrelapsers on 17 of these 21 variables—the 4 exceptions being *LOE-P* (Level of Expectations—Patient), *FTA-P* (Free-Time Activities—Patient), *Str-P*, and *Str-I.*

Among the five variables which discriminated significantly or near-significantly, the patient as respondent is represented only in the judgmental category: Relapsers were more dissatisfied with themselves, with reference both to socially-expected activities and free-time activities. In contrast, for informants there was one discriminating KAS variable in each of the three content categories: psychopathological, social, judgmental. As appraised by informants, relapsers at Month 12 were more anxious than nonrelapsers and were somewhat less effective in their social functioning. As indicated by the adjusted *LOE-I* means, informants reported having expected less of relapsers than of nonrelapsers (in terms of social behavior at Month 12) when they had first left Spring Grove and entered our study—a realistic outlook, as gauged by the *SEA-I* discrepancy. Thus in the general area of socially constructive behavior the discriminating patient-reported measures are those having to do with satisfaction, while informant-reported discriminations pertain to actual social performance and to the observers' prior expectations for that performance.

All in all, with initial differences taken into account, the evidence in Table III-7 that relapsers may have ended the year with greater net disturbance than nonrelapsers is suggestive but not convincing. Evidence from another source, however, pointed up more decisively a comparatively deteriorating course of adjustment for relapsers. It was based on a single comprehensive index of year-long adjustment outcome, using as raw input data the global adjustment scores for Months 1 and 12 (Appendix O). For each patient in the anchor-months cohort, an "outcome index" was calculated, using the traditional simple arithmetical change score but with a built-in correction for individual differences in Month-1 global adjustment (Appendix Q). On the outcome index, patients scoring 500 or more are by definition classified as having had a relatively "favorable" course of adjustment, while those scoring 499 or less are classified "unfavorable." As graphed in Figure III-3, obtained outcome indexes ranged from 505 to 667 in the favorable group ($N$ = 53, 56 per cent) and from 231 to 499 in the unfavorable group ($N$ = 41, 44 per cent); the two groups combined averaged 500, S.D. 100. It was then possible to subdivide both the 73 nonrelapsers and the 21 relapsers by favorable *vs.* unfavorable outcomes. The resulting four-cell contingency table showed the following percentages for unfavorable outcome: nonrelapsers, 37 per cent (27

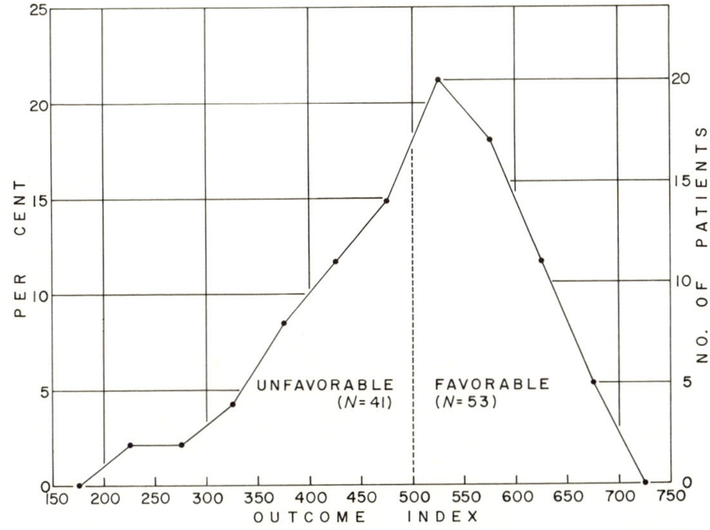


Figure III-3. Distribution and dichotomization of outcome index scores.

cases); relapsers, 67 per cent (14 cases); all cohort patients, 44 per cent (41 cases). The outcome difference, favoring nonrelapsers almost two to one, was significant at the .02 level ($\chi^2 = 5.84$). The same comparison, when made by *t* test, was significant at the .10 level: Nonrelapsers had an average outcome index of 509, S.D. 100, while relapsers averaged 469, S.D. 94. Rehospitalization during the year does, then, seem to have involved a comparatively unhealthy course of adjustment.

## *Life Situation*

In longitudinally comparing nonrelapsers with relapsers, our method was basically the same for life-situation variables as for adjustment variables. Analogous compilations of raw data were undertaken, and the same strictures apply to interpretation of results. In addition, three provisos peculiar to the life-situation comparisons should be noted. (1) Data analyses were nonparametric. (2) For some items data were missing (Appendix R). (3) It was not possible to test for differences on every variable at every month: missing data, in conjunction with missed tests and skewed distributions of some of the obtained data, reduced the number of analyses from the possible total of 480 (40 variables x 12 months) to an actual total of 328, slightly over two-thirds of 480.[4] Table III-8 summarizes the results of all tests significant at or beyond the .05 level.

As compared with the adjustment variables, life-situation variables discriminated much less effectively between nonrelapsers and relapsers. The tabulated results cover only 21 out of the 328 sig-

[4]Commentary on results is focused on those variables and months for which significance tests *could* be made. For patient and informant variables alike, about two-thirds of all comparisons were testable. In three of the four life-situation areas–home and family, work and homemaking, and stress–about three-fourths of the comparisons were testable, while in the treatment area only one-half could be analyzed. Seven of the 40 life-situation variables eluded analysis either at every single month or at 11 months out of 12:

Step-, in-law children in home;
Drug: how long used (both respondents);
Drug: amount used (both respondents);
Stress: Social and recreational (both respondents).

Not more than four monthly comparisons proved impossible to test in the case of any of those variables showing significant differences (Table III-8).

*Table III-8. Significant Monthly Differences in Life Situation between Nonrelapsers and Relapsers (Complete Cases Only)*

| Item | Respondent | Significant Results | | Difference[a] | |
|---|---|---|---|---|---|
| | | Month No. | $p$ | Nonrelapsers | Relapsers |
| Home and family: | | | | | |
| Type of home | Patient | 1, 2, 3, 4 | .05 to .025 | More in conjugal home | More in parental or other type home |
| Work and homemaking: | | | | | |
| Employment: duration | Patient | 10, 11, 12 | .02 to .001 | Longer time on job | Shorter time on job |
| Employment: duration | Informant | 10, 11, 12 | .01 to .001 | Longer time on job | Shorter time on job |
| Breadwinner contribution[b] | Informant | 12 | .025 | Greater contribution | Less contribution |
| Homemaker responsibility[b] | Patient | 1, 2, 3, 11 | .05 to .02 | Greater responsibility | Less responsibility |
| Homemaker responsibility[b] | Informant | 4 | .05 | Greater responsibility | Less responsibility |
| Treatment: | | | | | |
| Where received | Patient | 12 | .025 | More treated "nowhere" | Fewer treated "nowhere" |
| Outlook for future | Patient | 12 | .02 | Fewer planning to continue or start | More planning to continue or start |
| Drug: how long prescribed[b] | Informant | 10, 12 | .05 | Fewer with drug all month | More with drug all month |
| Stress: | | | | | |
| Marital and sexual | Patient | 10 | .05 | Lower incidence of stress | Higher incidence of stress |

[a]The indicated differences were observed at every month where significant results were found.

[b]Some cases excluded; see Appendix R.

nificance tests, or 1 out of 16. Are these results mere chance fluctuations? Certainly that suspicion is tenable; nonetheless, all four life-situation areas are represented, and a consistent (apparently nonrandom) pattern is implicit in the "difference" columns. In the areas of home and family, and work and homemaking, nonrelapsers uniformly demonstrated the more mature social functioning. (Undoubtedly, the work and homemaking variables are appreciably correlated with KAS measures of social functioning such as those shown in Table III-6; we have not investigated these correlations per se.)

Significant discriminations in the area of treatment are seen only toward the end of the year, when relapsers who had returned home were planning or receiving aftercare more often than nonrelapsers. That such differences emerge only late in the year may reflect increased clinical effort to prevent further repetitions of hospitalizations: we have already seen that sicker patients tended more often to have drugs at Month 1 (Table III-5), and that it was relapsers who were sicker throughout the posthospital year (Table III-6). Thus a distinctive triad appears to have been at work in the relapsers' course of adjustment: deteriorating adjustment, frequent outpatient treatment, and frequent rehospitalization. In this context there is room for doubt that outpatient treatment was fulfilling its mission of preventing rehospitalization.

Taking all of the life-situation results together (Table III-8), we note that significant differences between nonrelapsers and relapsers occurred with some frequency during the early months 1 through 4, not at all for the mid-year months 5 through 9, and most frequently at the terminal months 10 through 12. Thus the period of greatest density for life-situation differences was roughly the same as for adjustment differences (Table III-6). Probably these end-of-year patterns are in part a reflection of rehospitalized patients' having returned to the community and, with their further eroded personal resources, rejoined the cohort of subjects undergoing monthly tests. In life situation, it is this kind of infiltration which seems to be reflected not only in the treatment differences (as we have already noted), but also in the superior employment record of nonrelapsers at Months 10, 11, and 12. Similarly, in adjustment (Table III-6) we may be witnessing, at least within a limited one-year span, a progressive demarcation between (1) patients with a relatively benign course of adjustment (nonrelapsers) and (2) patients whose illness is following an inexorably deteriorating course, despite their having received both inpatient and outpatient treatment (relapsers). The relapsers' deterioration may actually have been aggravated or induced by rehospitalization, notwithstanding the therapeutic intent of inpatient treatment (Honigfeld and Gillis, 1967).

Neither patient nor informant emerges as a superior discriminator in Table III-8: each respondent contributes roughly his proportionate share to the significant results. The same cannot be said for the four major life-situation areas: the work and homemaking area is overrepresented, while stress is markedly underrepresented. (Life-situation area comparisons will be made in this manner throughout the report. They are based on the same tabulation method as that described for the three content categories of adjustment variables.)

## RELATIONS BETWEEN LIFE SITUATION AND GLOBAL ADJUSTMENT

Life situation and adjustment are molar ongoing processes—the former being heavily weighted with environmental forces and the latter with behavioral. It is imperative not only to trace their fluctuations throughout the posthospital year, but also to elucidate some of their intricate interrelationships. We began by using one-way analyses of variance to test concurrent relations between life situation and global adjustment at anchor months 1 and 12.

### *Concurrent Relations: Month 1*

Of the 40 standard life situation variables, 15 (48 per cent) were significantly related to KAS global adjustment at Month 1, at or beyond the .05 level, in the total sample of 139 participants. As shown in Table III-9, each of the four major life-situation areas was represented by one or more significant findings.

In the "home and family" area, adjustment was poorest among those patients whose closest affiliation was with parent(s). Conversely, spouse-affiliated patients were consistently the best ad-

*Table III-9. Concurrent Life Situation Variables Related Significantly ($p \leq .05$) to KAS Global Adjustment at Month 1 (Participants, N = 139)*

| Life Situation | | KAS Global Adjustment | |
|---|---|---|---|
| Item | Respondent, *N* | Mean | S.D. |
| Home and family | | | |
| Type of home ($p < .005$): | Patient | | |
| Conjugal | 87 | 4.64 | 1.17 |
| Parental | 32 | 3.60* | 1.19 |
| All other | 20 | 3.94 | 1.63 |
| Closest living relative ($p < .01$): | Patient | | |
| Spouse | 103 | 4.48 | 1.26 |
| Parent, child, or sibling | 36 | 3.77* | 1.38 |
| Informant ($p < .01$): | Informant | | |
| Spouse | 69 | 4.56 | 1.16 |
| Parent | 28 | 3.46* | 1.21 |
| Son or daughter | 12 | 4.53 | 1.02 |
| Sibling | 14 | 4.45 | 1.28 |
| All other | 16 | 4.33 | 1.77 |
| Father living or deceased ($p < .025$): | Patient | | |
| Living | 62 | 3.98* | 1.41 |
| Deceased (1 case Uncertain) | 77 | 4.55 | 1.20 |
| Work and homemaking | | | |
| Busiest single work week ($p < .01$):[a] | Patient | | |
| Less than full time | 8 | 3.24* | 1.99 |
| Full time or more | 22 | 5.09 | 1.18 |
| Busiest single work week ($p < .005$):[a] | Informant | | |
| Less than full time | 7 | 3.02* | 2.03 |
| Full time or more | 22 | 5.03 | 1.17 |
| Breadwinner contribution ($p < .001$):[a] | Informant | | |
| No contribution | 85 | 4.28 | 1.21 |
| Less than major | 30 | 3.91* | 1.56 |
| Sole or major breadwinner | 13 | 5.71 | 0.65 |
| Homemaker responsibility ($p < .01$):[a] | Patient | | |
| None, self only, or shared | 41 | 3.82* | 1.51 |
| Sole responsibility | 54 | 4.58 | 1.15 |
| Homemaker responsibility ($p < .005$):[a] | Informant | | |
| None, self only, or shared | 42 | 3.81* | 1.59 |
| Sole responsibility | 53 | 4.64 | 1.01 |
| Treatment | | | |
| Outlook for future ($p < .025$): | Patient | | |
| No plan to continue or start | 29 | 4.81 | 1.31 |
| Plan to continue or start | 110 | 4.16* | 1.28 |

*Table III-9. (Continued)*

| Life Situation | | KAS Global Adjustment | |
|---|---|---|---|
| Item | Respondent, $N$ | Mean | S.D. |
| Stress | | | |
| "Bad" event(s) during month ($p < .005$): | Patient | | |
| One or more | 50 | 3.84* | 1.43 |
| None | 89 | 4.55 | 1.19 |
| Interpersonal stress ($p < .005$): | Patient | | |
| Some | 46 | 3.78* | 1.42 |
| None | 93 | 4.55 | 1.20 |
| Marital and sexual stress ($p < .01$): | Informant | | |
| Some | 35 | 3.76* | 1.44 |
| None | 104 | 4.48 | 1.24 |
| Economic and domestic stress ($p < .001$): | Patient | | |
| Some | 41 | 3.71* | 1.31 |
| None | 98 | 4.54 | 1.26 |
| Occupational stress ($p < .025$): | Informant | | |
| Some | 44 | 3.91* | 1.45 |
| None | 95 | 4.47 | 1.23 |

*Note*: All significance tests based on *F*. Asterisk * indicates worst mean subgroup score for each life-situation item.

[a]Some cases excluded; see Appendix R.

justed. To the extent that informants contributed to the global adjustment score (Appendix O), there may have been slanting of these results by way of favorable KAS reporting from spouse-informants *vs.* comparatively unfavorable reporting by parent-informants. Even when this is discounted, however, the results still seem to reflect immaturity and dependency on the part of the parent-affiliated patient. It may also have been that parents, in their interactions with patients, generated a less wholesome or supportive interpersonal climate than did spouses. At any rate, parents figured more decisively in adjustment than did children: none of the three variables pertaining to children yielded a significant relationship with global adjustment.

The "work and homemaking" area was the one proportionately most heavily saturated with significant relations to global adjustment. Duration of employment (both respondents), expressed as a proportion of Month-1 time, is the only variable in this area not represented in Table III-9. All of the work and homemaking items overlap considerably in content some of the items in KAS *SEA-P* and *SEA-I*; and since both of these KAS variables are used in the global adjustment formula, such significant relationships as were found were partly predetermined. Hence these findings are less fruitful for inference and interpretation than are those in the other life-situation areas. At any rate, the most poorly adjusted patients at Month 1 were usually those who were unemployed or working only part-time, and those (females) who were carrying less than major responsibility as homemakers. The "breadwinner contribution" item exhibits an interesting nonlinearity in its relation to global adjustment: Those patients who were making "no contribution" were on the average better, not worse, adjusted than those whose contribution was rated by the informant as "less than major." Conceivably, the "less than major" breadwinner suffered from a conflict in this area which for better or for worse had been resolved both by the "sole or major" breadwinners and by the "no contribution" patients.

Only one of the nine treatment variables was significantly related to global adjustment. Complementing previous findings, it was the sicker patients who were receiving or about to begin aftercare. Treatment in certain facilities, or nowhere, was not differentially related to severity of illness; nor were any of the drug treatment items, nor the receipt of any treatment other than chemotherapy.

In the stress area, there were 16 items to be analyzed: the two general stress items "good" and "bad", and the 6 specific stress items representing sectors of the environment—each item having been answered by both respondents, patient and informant. Five of the 16 analyses of variance showed stress to have been positively associated with poor global adjustment at Month 1.[5] Only three of the eight stress items are not represented by either respondent in Table III-9: "good" event(s) during month; social and recreational stress; and physical health. It is at this particular juncture in our entire series of data analyses that stress makes perhaps

[5]These results, together with the stress findings in Table III-10, may be compared with the roughly analogous intercorrelations among stress index scores and KAS scores presented in Appendix M.

its most decisive appearance, in terms of meaningful and significant relations. It is possible that environmental stress was highest at Month 1, when all patients had freshly returned home from the hospital and were coping with readjustments to home and community; later results support this proposition, as does Pao's clinical study of schizophrenic mothers' early posthospital domestic problems (Pao, 1960). It is also possible that, with succeeding months, patients who remained at home were able to adapt more effectively to external pressures as they persisted or arose anew. Especially relevant to this outlook are the theoretical speculations of Dohrenwend and Dohrenwend (1965). In a careful appraisal of validity problems in psychiatric field studies, they surveyed about 20 major research publications. One of their prime conclusions was that many of the subjects who were rated mentally ill in these researches may actually have been normals, suffering only from transitory reactions to environmental stress. (For our purposes, we may substitute here: psychiatric patients responding to stress via exacerbation of illness.) They went on to postulate: "If the symptoms normal persons develop when exposed to stressors disappear spontaneously on removal of the stressors, then it is clear that these symptoms indicate situationally induced response rather than self-perpetuating pathology in the individual. The weight of the evidence is that spontaneous recovery is frequent." Again, applying this notion to our patients: They, as well as normals, may have been able to respond more effectively to stress *after* its initial impact at Month 1. Such a development, facilitated by the actual lessening of stress as later reported, would account for the Month-1 concentration of stress's relations to global adjustment.

A final observation concerning Table III-9 has to do with the proportionate contributions of the two independent respondents to the obtained significant results. There was no difference whatever: of the 24 patient items and 16 informant items, equal proportions achieved inclusion in the table.

*Concurrent Relations: Month 12*

At Month 12, only nine of the 40 life-situation variables were by one-way analysis of variance significantly related to global adjustment. Thus the rate of significant results dropped from 38 per cent at Month 1 to 22 per cent at Month 12. We must here again consider the possibility that chance was the prime determinant of results. However, the directions of the mean global adjustment differences suggest otherwise; and, comparing results from one set of analyses to another as we can now begin to do, we can see emerging patterns of clinically meaningful relationship which also contraindicate mere chance fluctuations in the significance tests.

Considering the four life-situation areas, there are revealing similarities and differences between Months 1 and 12 (Tables III-9 and III-10). The Month-12 home-and-family situation has no representation whatever among the significant discriminators, and the representation of stress is quite negligible; apparently, in both areas, patients at Month 12 have had time to come to terms with these aspects of the environment, at least to the extent that severity of illness no longer covaries with them.

The work-and-homemaking area maintained (and even increased) at Month 12 the discriminating ascendancy it had shown at Month 1. Item by item the two patterns of findings are not identical, but at the year's end it was still the busiest patients who were least sick.

As regards treatment, we have already seen in Table III-8 that discriminations between nonrelapsers and relapsers were concentrated at the end of the year. A quite similar trend is seen in the relation between treatment and global adjustment (Tables III-9 and III-10). It is the terminal period, not the initial one, where treatment is decisively related to severity of illness, and it is clearly the sicker patients who are being treated. (The sickest are attending the Spring Grove Outpatient Clinic, though they are on the average very little sicker than patients treated elsewhere.) To conclude that treatment during the year has made patients worse would be improper, though there is certainly no evidence that it has yielded improvement. Most likely, the end-of-year treatment discriminations stem from selective patient movement, with improved patients leaving treatment and worsening patients entering or resuming it.

The almost total lack of significant relations between stress and global adjustment at Month 12 contrasts strikingly with the previously discussed Month-1 findings (Table III-9).

*Table III-10. Concurrent Life Situation Variables Related Significantly ($p \leq .05$) to KAS Global Adjustment at Month 12 ($N = 94$)*

| Life Situation | | KAS Global Adjustment | |
|---|---|---|---|
| Item | Respondent, *N* | Mean | S.D. |
| Work and homemaking | | | |
| Employment: duration ($p < .05$): | Patient | | |
| No part of month | 58 | 4.45 | 1.23 |
| Part of month | 9 | 4.12* | 1.44 |
| All month | 27 | 5.14 | 1.13 |
| Employment: duration ($p < .05$): | Informant | | |
| No part of month | 60 | 4.36* | 1.31 |
| Part of month | 8 | 4.85 | 0.73 |
| All month | 26 | 5.14 | 1.15 |
| Homemaker responsibility ($p < .05$):[a] | Patient | | |
| None, self only, or shared | 17 | 3.99* | 1.28 |
| Sole responsibility | 47 | 4.76 | 1.25 |
| Homemaker responsibility ($p < .005$):[a] | Informant | | |
| None, self only, or shared | 21 | 3.81* | 1.33 |
| Sole responsibility | 43 | 4.91 | 1.12 |
| Treatment | | | |
| Where received ($p < .05$): | Patient | | |
| Nowhere (not in treatment) | 28 | 5.20 | 1.17 |
| Spring Grove Outpatient Clinic | 36 | 4.26* | 1.11 |
| Public clinic other than Spring Grove | 10 | 4.52 | 1.18 |
| All other: private doctor, etc. | 20 | 4.50 | 1.43 |
| Outlook for future treatment ($p < .025$): | Patient | | |
| No plan to continue or start | 35 | 5.03 | 1.20 |
| Plan to continue or start | 59 | 4.37* | 1.25 |
| Drug: how long prescribed ($p < .025$): | Patient | | |
| None or part of month | 35 | 5.03 | 1.24 |
| All month | 59 | 4.37* | 1.23 |
| Drug: how long prescribed ($p < .01$):[a] | Informant | | |
| None or part of month | 37 | 5.06 | 1.21 |
| All month | 56 | 4.31* | 1.23 |
| Stress | | | |
| Physical health stress ($p < .025$): | Informant | | |
| Some | 24 | 4.07* | 1.46 |
| None | 70 | 4.80 | 1.15 |

*Note:* All significance tests based on *F*. Asterisk * indicates worst mean subgroup score for each life-situation item.

[a]Some cases excluded; see Appendix R.

As was true for Month 1, neither patient nor informant monopolized significant results as respondent at Month 12 (Table III-10). Moreover, detailed inspection of frequencies and mean scores in Tables III-9 and III-10 discloses indirect evidence that patients and informants agreed rather closely in their independent reports on matching items. (See also Appendix M, Table M-2, row 1.)

*Changes in Life Situation as Related to Outcome*

In the anchor-months cohort, were there changes in life situation during the posthospital year that were systematically related to favorable *vs.* unfavorable course of adjustment? For each of the 40 life-situation variables, we sought to answer this question by: (1) classifying patients as to (a) change *vs.* no change in comparison of Months 1 and 12 and (b) direction of change if any, and (2) testing for differences between favorables and unfavorables within this schema. Testable contingency tables could be developed only for 17 of the 40 variables in question. The remaining 23 were lost to missing data (Appendix R) and/or skewed distributions with zero frequencies in some cells.

In order to manage the data on this basis, we dichotomized each life situation item not originally so structured (thus undesirably but unavoidably obscuring some potentially important changes): for example, employment was reduced to "all or some of month" *vs.* "none." The two halves of each such dichotomy were designated "Status 1" and "Status 2." Each of the 94 anchor-months cohort patients was then allocated to one of four categories: (1) Status 1 at both months; (2) Status 2 at both months; (3) Status 1 at Month 1, Status 2 at Month 12; (4) Status 2 at Month 1, Status 1 at Month 12. Eight-cell contingency tables were based on these four categories, each subdivided to contain patients with favorable and unfavorable course of adjustment (Figure III-3).

From the 17 completed analyses, no relations significant at the .05 level were found between life-situation changes and outcome. On two life-situation items, borderline differences ($p < .10$) were found; all 94 cohort cases were represented in both of these analyses.

Employment *vs.* unemployment, during Month 1 as compared with Month 12 (informant's report), discriminated in the plausible direction, showing differences mainly in two of the four status categories. Among the favorables, 21 per cent who began the year unemployed were working at Month 12; the same was true for only 7 per cent of unfavorables. Patients who were uncmployed at both anchor months constituted 57 per cent of the favorable outcome groups as against 73 per cent of the unfavorable.

Marital and sexual stress (patient's report) was the second item showing a borderline outcome difference. Comparative proportions in the two outcome groups were in accord with our working hypothesis concerning stress. Twenty-one per cent of the favorables reported marital and sexual stress at Month 1 but not at Month 12, while only 5 per cent of the unfavorables had this pattern of change. The obverse pattern–negative for stress in this area at Month 1, but positive at Month 12–held true for 11 per cent of favorables and 17 per cent of unfavorables.[6]

Meager results such as these give pause for candid, self-searching reflections on methodology. We strongly suspect that in this subarea of investigation (and in not a few of our others as well) psychosocial forces were at work more potently than we were able to register them. Even at some points within our own study design, tighter and more effective data analyses might have been possible–given unlimited time, which one never has. Certainly future studies of such processes, less involved than our own in trials and demonstrations of relatively new methods, can employ phenomenological nets with stronger strands and smaller meshes.

[6]By life-situation area, the 17 testable items (including the two discussed) were:
Home and Family–0 items out of total of 8

Work and Homemaking–4 out of 7:
- Employment: duration (both respondents)
- Busiest single work week (both respondents)

Treatment–1 out of 9:
- Treatment other than drug

Stress–12 out of 16 (6 items, both respondents):
- "Good" event(s) during month
- "Bad" event(s) during month
- Interpersonal
- Marital and sexual
- Economic and domestic
- Physical health

## NONRELAPSERS' COURSE OF ADJUSTMENT

The 51 complete cases who achieved nonrelapser classification constituted an elite in three respects. They were by circumstance and motivation available for study; they and their informants missed only 2.7 per cent of the 1,224 individual monthly evaluations (17 patient sessions and 17 informant sessions were missed); and they remained unrehospitalized for the entire study year. By virtue of these distinctions, the cadre of "complete nonrelapsers" afforded unique opportunity for fine-grained depiction and study of course of adjustment. Differential trends from month to month on each of the 26 adjustment variables could be delineated, and an attempt could be made to answer the paramount question: On the average, did these comparatively successful patients improve, worsen, or simply not change appreciably during the posthospital year?

Tables III-11 and III-12 describe the patients in terms of the standard background variables. Their mean age was 42.2, S.D. 12.7; education averaged 10.8 years, S.D. 3.0.

Because of the various lacunae in our data on participants, the most intensive analyses (and, often, those bearing on the most crucial questions) must tend to be self-limited to smaller subsamples. Accordingly, to devote special attention to the "complete nonrelapser" group involves considerable sacrificing of sample representativeness so as to focus on important investigative issues. Completes differ somewhat from other participants, and rather markedly from nonparticipants (see Chapter II and Appendix N); furthermore, nonrelapsers are in many respects unlike relapsers (as specified directly above and in Chapter V). Cognizance of the complete nonrelapsers' characteristic features is of course essential for effective understanding of the results to be presented on this group.[7]

[7]Complete nonrelapsers had a mean outcome index (523, S.D. 93) somewhat better than that of the 22 semi-complete nonrelapsers (476, S.D. 108); the difference was of borderline significance, $p < .10$. Further: in the anchor-months cohort we have already seen that outcome indexes were likewise somewhat more favorable for nonrelapsers than for relapsers. Thus, in singling out complete nonrelapsers for these analyses, we are excluding participants whose course of adjustment, as measured by the outcome index, was probably slightly inferior.

*Table III-11. Complete Nonrelapsers (N = 51): Distributions for Demographic Background Variables*

| Variable | *N* | Per Cent |
|---|---|---|
| Age: | | |
| 18 to 29 | 8 | 16 |
| 30 to 39 | 13 | 25 |
| 40 to 49 | 14 | 27 |
| 50 to 59 | 10 | 20 |
| 60 to 69 | 5 | 10 |
| 70 to 74 | 1 | 2 |
| Sex: | | |
| Male | 15 | 29 |
| Female | 36 | 71 |
| Marital status: | | |
| Single | 7 | 14 |
| Married | 38 | 74 |
| Widowed | 3 | 6 |
| Separated | 3 | 6 |
| Divorced | 0 | 0 |
| No. of children: | | |
| None | 11 | 22 |
| 1 | 7 | 14 |
| 2 | 14 | 27 |
| 3 or 4 | 15 | 29 |
| 5 or more | 4 | 8 |
| Religion: | | |
| Catholic | 16 | 31 |
| Protestant | 32 | 63 |
| Jewish | 3 | 6 |
| Years of education: | | |
| 4 to 8 | 14 | 27 |
| 9 to 11 | 12 | 24 |
| 12 | 14 | 27 |
| 13 to 19 | 11 | 22 |
| Occupation: | | |
| Never employed | 31 | 61 |
| Professional and managerial | 4 | 8 |
| Clerical and sales | 4 | 8 |
| Service | 3 | 6 |
| Agriculture, fishing, and forestry | 0 | 0 |
| Skilled labor | 3 | 6 |
| Semi-skilled labor | 4 | 8 |
| Unskilled labor | 2 | 4 |

*Table III-12. Complete Nonrelapsers (N = 51): Distributions for Clinical Background Variables*

| Variable | *N* | Per Cent |
|---|---|---|
| Number of hospitalizations prior to last: | | |
| None (first admission) | 19 | 37 |
| One | 14 | 27 |
| Two or three | 9 | 18 |
| Four or five | 3 | 6 |
| Six or more | 6 | 12 |
| Years hospitalized prior to last admission: | | |
| None (first admission) | 32 | 63 |
| One-half or less | 0 | 0 |
| One | 10 | 20 |
| Two to fifteeen | 6 | 12 |
| Unknown | 3 | 6 |
| Months hospitalized during last admission: | | |
| One or less | 17 | 33 |
| Two | 11 | 22 |
| Three | 9 | 18 |
| Four to six | 6 | 12 |
| Seven to seventy-five | 8 | 16 |
| Final hospital diagnosis: | | |
| Schizophrenic reaction (all types) | 22 | 43 |
| Psychoses other than schizophrenia | 14 | 27 |
| Psychoneurotic disorders | 12 | 24 |
| Personality disorders | 3 | 6 |
| Type of release from hospital: | | |
| Convalescent leave | 42 | 82 |
| Discharge with doctor's consent | 9 | 18 |

## **Trend Analysis: Statistical Procedure*

In psychology, the problem of measuring and evaluating change is as persistent as it is fraught with pitfalls. Statisticians have expounded procedures for trend analysis along with cautions and limitations (Edwards, 1960, pp. 224-253; McNemar, 1962, pp. 346-361). Statistically oriented researchers have conscientiously sought solutions for general and special problems (Harris, 1963). Other investigators, more clinically committed, have devised procedures ingeniously suited to research situations not unlike our own (Engelhardt, Freedman, Hankoff, Mann, and Margolis, 1963).

On our 51 subjects, 12 monthly measurements were available on each of the 26 adjustment variables. The statistical approach chosen as most suitable, and least subject to artifact and impaired validity in assessing change in adjustment, was a modification of conventional trend analysis–developed and computerized in our own Research Department and originally intended for use in controlled chemotherapy research. Its authors explained:

> Our interest lies in the *trend* of the . . . means, and not merely whether or not these means display significant heterogeneity. Hence, we are interested in calculating the regression (slope) of the column means over time and determining the statistical significance of any resulting linear and/or curvilinear regressions. . . . In our opinion, an acceptable solution . . . is to calculate, by the method of orthogonal polynomials, the linear and nonlinear (quadratic, cubic, etc.) regression components for each individual subject's measurements *separately*. . . . For each component, the group mean and its standard error can be calculated and the mean tested for significance (from zero) by means of the customary *t* test . . . . A linear trend that significantly departs from the horizontal is self-explanatory; a quadratic trend is somewhat concave or convex; and a cubic trend is rather *S*-shaped. . . . The time intervals between observational points [must be] equal. . . . Data [must] be available at each observational point on each subject. . . . Provided the missing observations are relatively few (not more than 5 per cent of the total) and rather randomly distributed, it is our opinion that little violence is done to the data if the simple expedient of averaging a subject's adjacent values to fill the missing space is adopted. (Shaffer, Forbes, and DeFelice, 1967.)

Averaging of adjacent KAS scores was used in our own data compilation where tests had been missed.

### *Main Results*

Here our primary interest was in the statistical significance and clinical direction of the 12-month *linear* trend for each adjustment variable. Did it differ significantly by *t* test from a hypothetical level line representing no change during the year? If so, was the change toward improvement, or worsening?[8]

Grossly, the trend analysis results indicated manifold significant improvement. Means and S.D.'s on which these results are based are presented in entirety in Appendix S. Table III-13 summarizes the longitudinal course for all adjustment variables and includes a composite index of change on each. Of the 26 variables, significant change in the direction of improvement was found on the following 16 at the .05, .01, or .001 level as indicated:

| *p* | *Variable* |
|---|---|
| KAS–Patient: | |
| .01 | Symptom Discomfort (*Sym*) |
| .01 | Satisfaction with Socially-Expected Activities (*SSA-P*) |
| .05 | Satisfaction with Free-Time Activities (*SFA-P*) |
| KAS–Informant: | |
| .01 | Negativism (*Neg*) |
| .01 | Helplessness (*Hel*) |
| .05 | Suspiciousness (*Sus*) |
| .001 | Anxiety (*Anx*) |
| .01 | Withdrawal and Retardation (*Wdl*) |
| .001 | General Psychopathology (*Psy*) |
| .001 | Nervousness (*Ner*) |
| .001 | Hyperactivity (*Hyp*) |
| .05 | Performance of Socially-Expected Activities (*SEA-I*) |
| .001 | Level of Expectations (*LOE-I*) |
| .001 | Satisfaction with Free-Time Activities (*SFA-I*) |
| Stress Index: | |
| .01 | Patient Stress (*Str-P*) |
| .01 | Informant Stress (*Str-I*) |

[8]In the strictly clinical symptomatic sense, the terms "improvement" and "worsening" obviously do not apply to the two stress indexes, nor to changes in expectations and satisfaction as measured by *LOE*, *SSA*, and *SFA* (both respondents). Especially in a longitudinal context, *LOE* is quite different from the other adjustment variables. At Month 7, for instance, informants completing the *LOE* form were being asked: "When the patient left Spring Grove seven months ago, to what extent did you *then expect him* to be performing these (itemized) socially-expected activities *at this time* (Month 7)?" Thus, disappointment is reflected when at a given month an *LOE* score is less favorable than the same respondent's *SEA* score. By the same token, disappointment is indicated by the *SSA* scale alone: The higher its score, the greater is the item-by-item discrepancy between reported behavior (*SEA*) and expected behavior (*LOE*).

*T* scores for the 24 KAS measures at Months 1 and 12 are presented in Appendix T, for use by others working with this instrument.

*Improvement: Real or Spurious?*

It is well known that test-retest effects can simulate "improvement" where actually there may have been little or none; in some instances even spurious "worsening" may occur (Windle, 1954; Windle, 1955). The possibility that test-retest effects are at work in our trend analysis results is indicated especially by outcome-index differences between complete nonrelapsers and their 22 semicomplete counterparts, who had repeated the KAS far less frequently during the study year (see footnote 7). Ultimately, we obviously cannot disentangle real change from spurious change; however, several aspects of the problem do merit scrutiny.[9]

There is other evidence in our results, circumstantial but interesting, which tends to contraindicate serious test-retest distortions. Patient and informant, as independent respondents, contributed in quite similar proportions to the above list of significant trend analysis results. We know of no good reason, however, to expect spurious test-retest "improvement" in the *informant's* KAS reports; on the contrary, professional observers when repeatedly evaluating drug-treated psychiatric inpatients have shown to laspe into a "plateau" effect—failing to perceive latter-day favorable change which is perceived by other raters with less previous exposure to the same patients (Michaux, Ota, Hanlon, and Kurland, 1963). Campbell (1963, p. 219) also recognizes such a phenomenon, which he terms "instrument decay," as a potential source of

[9]The same interpretive complication applies to other outcome index comparisons already reported in this chapter, insofar as the groups in question differed as to frequency of repeated tests. This would include not only completes *vs.* semicompletes, but also nonrelapsers *vs.* relapsers—since relapsers missed testing legitimately during their rehospitalization months.

Test-retest effects in clinical research should not be thought of as limited to practice effects in test-taking. Test-taking may induce in the subject actual change in the characteristic being measured. Campbell (1963, p. 219) notes that "Such reactive effects can be expected whenever the testing process is in itself a stimulus to change rather than a passive record of behavior. Thus in an experiment on therapy for weight control, the initial weigh-in might in itself be a stimulus to weight reduction, even without the therapeutic treatment." Examiners in our project became convinced that just such quasi-therapeutic improvement tendencies did develop in some patients.

*Table III-13. Selected Results from 12-Month Trend Analysis of Adjustment Variables (Complete Nonrelapsers, N = 51)*

| Variable | Symbol | Mean | | | Average Change[a] | |
|---|---|---|---|---|---|---|
| | | Month 1 | Month 6 | Month 12 | Raw | *T* |
| KAS–Patient only: | | | | | | |
| Symptom discomfort | *Sym* | 22.7 | 17.5 | 13.2 | -5.5 | -2.8 |
| KAS–Patient (see also Informant below): | | | | | | |
| Performance of Socially-Expected Activities | *SEA-P* | 36.4 | 36.8 | 37.4 | 0.4 | 0.8[b] |
| Level of Expectations | *LOE-P* | 37.3 | 39.0 | 38.5 | 1.4 | 3.0[b] |
| Satisfaction with Socially-Expected Activities | *SSA-P* | 7.5 | 7.3 | 6.0 | -0.3 | -0.4 |
| Free-Time Activities | *FTA-P* | 47.6 | 47.4 | 46.8 | -0.3 | -0.5 |
| Satisfaction with Free-Time Activities | *SFA-P* | 29.9 | 29.2 | 27.6 | -1.3 | -2.3 |
| KAS–Informant only: | | | | | | |
| Belligerence | *Bel* | 4.5 | 4.3 | 4.4 | -0.2 | -2.2 |
| Verbal Expansiveness | *Exp* | 6.2 | 6.0 | 6.1 | -0.2 | -0.9 |
| Negativism | *Neg* | 12.1 | 11.3 | 11.1 | -0.8 | -3.0 |
| Helplessness | *Hel* | 5.7 | 5.1 | 5.0 | -0.6 | -3.3 |
| Suspiciousness | *Sus* | 4.9 | 4.5 | 4.6 | -0.4 | -2.5 |
| Anxiety | *Anx* | 7.7 | 6.7 | 6.4 | -1.0 | -3.8 |
| Withdrawal and Retardation | *Wdl* | 9.4 | 9.0 | 8.3 | -0.6 | -2.5 |
| General Psychopathology | *Psy* | 33.8 | 31.3 | 30.5 | -2.6 | -3.7 |
| Nervousness | *Ner* | 7.6 | 6.8 | 6.1 | -1.1 | -4.9 |
| Confusion | *Con* | 3.4 | 3.1 | 3.3 | -0.3 | -2.3 |
| Bizarreness | *Biz* | 5.7 | 5.5 | 5.6 | -0.1 | -0.8 |
| Hyperactivity | *Hyp* | 4.7 | 3.9 | 3.7 | -0.8 | -6.2 |
| Emotional Stability | *Sta* | 30.5 | 30.8 | 30.9 | 0.6 | 1.4[b] |

| | | | | | | |
|---|---|---|---|---|---|---|
| KAS–Informant (see also Patient above): | | | | | | |
| Performance of Socially-Expected Activities | *SEA-I* | 35.5 | 36.7 | 36.7 | 1.1 | 2.4[b] |
| Level of Expectations | *LOE-I* | 34.3 | 37.0 | 37.6 | 3.1 | 6.2[b] |
| Satisfaction with Socially-Expected Activities | *SSA-I* | 4.6 | 5.9 | 6.3 | 1.6 | 2.7 |
| Free-Time Activities | *FTA-I* | 49.1 | 47.5 | 47.9 | -1.5 | -3.3 |
| Satisfaction with Free-Time Activities | *SFA-I* | 28.8 | 27.5 | 26.2 | -1.6 | -3.7 |
| Stress Index: | | | | | | |
| Patient Stress | *Str-P* | 15.5 | 14.8 | 12.4 | -1.6 | -1.2 |
| Informant Stress | *Str-I* | 17.3 | 14.0 | 12.2 | -4.0 | -2.9 |

[a]Average change is the difference between the Month-1 mean and the composite mean of all scores for Months 2 through 12. Raw-score values are shown at the left; in the *T* column they are converted to *T* scores based on the complete nonrelapsers' Month-1 S.D.'s (not shown here). For most variables, a negative average change means better adjustment during Months 2 through 12; exceptions are noted in footnote b.

[b]For these five variables only, high raw scores indicate relatively *good* adjustment; hence the positive average changes mean better adjustment during Months 2 through 12.

experimental error: "Where human observers are used . . . processes of learning, fatiguing, etc., within the observers will produce . . . differences in their successive reports. . . . If essays are being graded, the grading standards may shift. . . . If classroom participation is being observed, then the observers may be more skillful or more blase on the second occasion."

By closely inspecting means on each variable for Months 1 through 6, and separately those for Months 7 through 12 (Appendix S), we could roughly test the two premises implicit in these considerations: (1) that test-retest effects were potently present—as would be suggested if patient means "improved" more consistently than informant means; and (2) that the repeated informant assessments exhibited the plateau effect, or "rater perseveration."[10] More specifically, the inspection revealed that, scale by scale during Months 2 . . . 6, 69 per cent of the patient means were better than at Month 1, while 92 per cent of the informant means were better. For the first half of the year, then, premise (1) was not supported; informants, who should be comparatively free of such effects, reported not *less* improvement than patients but *more*. Premise (2) did gain support from the same approach when applied to the second half of the year, where rater perseveration might have been expected. Here the informant means did not maintain their higher rate of registering favorable change. During Months 8 through 12, 42 per cent of them were better than at Month 7, while the corresponding patient rate was 63 per cent, changing little from the first half-year period. Despite the informants' apparent plateau tendency, however—and despite their presumably being less susceptible than patients to test-retest "improvement" effects—their trend analyses yielded, as noted, numerous results significantly indicating favorable linear change. We tentatively conclude from these observations that, while test-retest effects were doubtless present in the trend analysis results (at least in the patient variables), those effects were not of such

[10]Infrequently, the informant role shifted from one individual to another (Appendix K, Table K-7). Presumably such shifts mitigated against plateau effects in the total body of data. We have not treated separately the cases where the person of the informant changed during the testing series.

magnitude as to rule out genuine improvement in the "complete nonrelapser" group.

Nor did the significant improvement trends appear to depend mainly on highly unfavorable starting levels measured in *T* score unit distances between Month-1 means and best possible scores. High initial levels were clearly not predominant among the 16 variables showing significant linear improvement, though they were observed for some variables.

## *Some General Tendencies*

For 9 of the remaining 10 adjustment variables, direction of change was favorable—as indicated both by average change (Table III-13) and by initial *vs.* end-of-year means. The one exception, *SSA-I* (Satisfaction with Socially-Expected Activities—Informant), will be discussed below; as with the other nine, its linear trend was nonsignificantly different from a level, changeless line extending from Month 1 to Month 12.

Among the 16 significant trends, psychopathological variables (Appendix P) were overrepresented—mainly because of the informant's contributions in this area. Judgmental variables appeared in normal proportion, while social variables were less in evidence than expected. The informant alone yielded a balanced representation of improvement across the three content categories; the patient's self-report reflected no significant improvement in the social area but was heavily weighted with judgmental scales. Again, then, the informant is the respondent who may have provided the more effective psychometric coverage; defensiveness and adverse self-preoccupation may have been distorting factors in the patient's reports on himself.

Two adjustment variables emerge as having been consistently sensitive in our major analyses dealing with course of adjustment: the patient judgmental variable *SFA-P* (Satisfaction with Free-time Activities—Patient) and the informant psychopathological variable *Anx*. In addition to registering improvement in the complete nonrelapsers, both variables have discriminated effectively between nonrelapsers and relapsers—not only longitudinally (Table

III-6) but also in terms of net change at year's end (Table III-7). (*Anx* was also psychometrically effective in the descriptive comparison with other patient groups, Figure II-1; *SFA-P* was not included in that comparison.)

In another posthospital study (Gordon, Rosenberg, and Morris, 1966), adult male schizophrenics were found to be less than normally active in recreation and to favor passive items such as watching television. It was concluded that many such patients needed recreational guidance. For our own patients, at least half of whom at every month were not gainfully employed, it is understandable how "satisfaction with free-time activities" could have been a major issue in adjustment. Moreover, it is noteworthy that trend analyses showed no significant improvement in actual participation in free-time activities as reported by either respondent on *FTA*.

As observed by the informant and reported on the KAS, the "anxious" patient was one who was easily and strangely frightened, who inordinately feared for present and future, and who verbalized his apprehensions, perhaps to the point of mentioning suicide. Judging from intercorrelations at Months 1 and 12 (Appendix M, Table M-1), this kind of anxiety was for the most part indigenously psychopathological and not highly related to concurrent social and environmental processes. It is interesting that *Anx* and *SFA-P* were among the few pairs of adjustment variables not significantly correlated with each other at either of the anchor months.

Figure III-4 depicts the complete nonrelapsers' initial and final status on all 26 adjustment variables. These graphs do not, of course, embody all of the data processed in the trend analyses, which took into account scores at every one of the 12 months. The informant's satisfaction with the patient's socially-expected activities here stands out as the only variable showing less favorable average status at Month 12 than at Month 1.

### *Socially-Expected Activities*

Three KAS patient scales, with counterparts in the informant form, deal with socially-expected activities. *SEA* measures actual

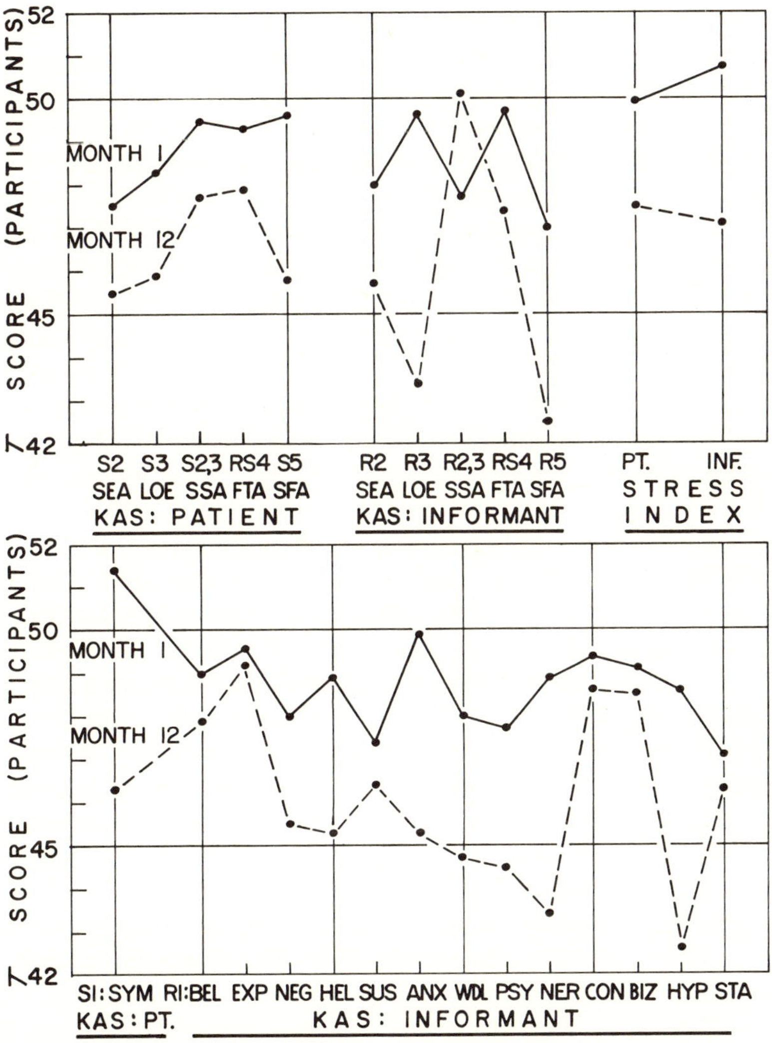


Figure III-4. Mean KAS and Stress Index scores of the complete nonrelapser group ($N = 51$) at the beginning and end of the posthospital year. The $T$ scale is based on the Month-1 scores of all participants ($N = 139$). To make high scores unfavorable on all scales, direction is reversed for KAS Socially-Expected Activities (S2 and R2: *SEA*), Level of Expectations (S3 and R3: *LOE*), and Stability (R1: *Sta*). Top graph shows scales common to patient and informant reports; bottom graph shows scales used only for one or the other of the two respondents.

performance; *LOE* measures expectations for the same behavioral items; and *SSA* measures discrepancy between reported performance and reported expectations. It is illuminating to take special note of the trend analysis findings on these three interlocking measures.

Let us first consider only the basic *SEA* measure as portrayed by raw-score means plotted for both respondents in Figure III-5. The smoothed best-fit lines are derived by the usual linear regression formula $Y = A + BX$. The linear trend for *SEA-P* (Performance of Socially-Expected Activities—Patient) barely missed significance at the .05 level ($t = 1.82$, $df = 50$, $p < .10$), while *SEA-I* with a slightly steeper slope did reach the .05 level ($t = 2.11$, $df = 50$).

Both raw-score curves exhibit interesting deviations from linearity. The *SEA-P* mean, but not the *SEA-I*, showed *worse* adjustment at Month 2 than at Month 1. Why? A clue is found in a candid comment from a patient who had finished the study: she admitted having withheld unfavorable information at Month 1 which she thereafter felt safe in revealing. Examining all other trend analysis means for the first two months (Appendix S, Table S-1), we find that five of the seven patient variables (including *SEA*) worsened here, while only one of the 19 informant variables did so—that one being *SSA-I*, which atypically continued to worsen at every succeeding month. In still another respect, then, Month 1 appears to have been a time of especially precarious security for the patient. Informant-reported stress supports this presumption: not only was *Str-I* highest at Month 1, but at no time did it decline more sharply than from Month 1 to Month 2 (Appendix S, Table S-1).

For the informant means (Figure III-5), one of the most jagged deviations from linearity occurs in the worsening upswing from Month 10 to Month 12. Indeed, improvement virtually vanishes from Month 8 onward. "Rater perseveration" or "instrument decay" appears prepotent here, especially in contrast with the orderly downward progression of corresponding monthly means in the patient graph.

Figure III-6 permits longitudinal comparison of patients with informants on all three of their matching KAS measures dealing with socially-expected activities. What is most revealing here, however, is to conjoin these comparisons with cross-comparisons

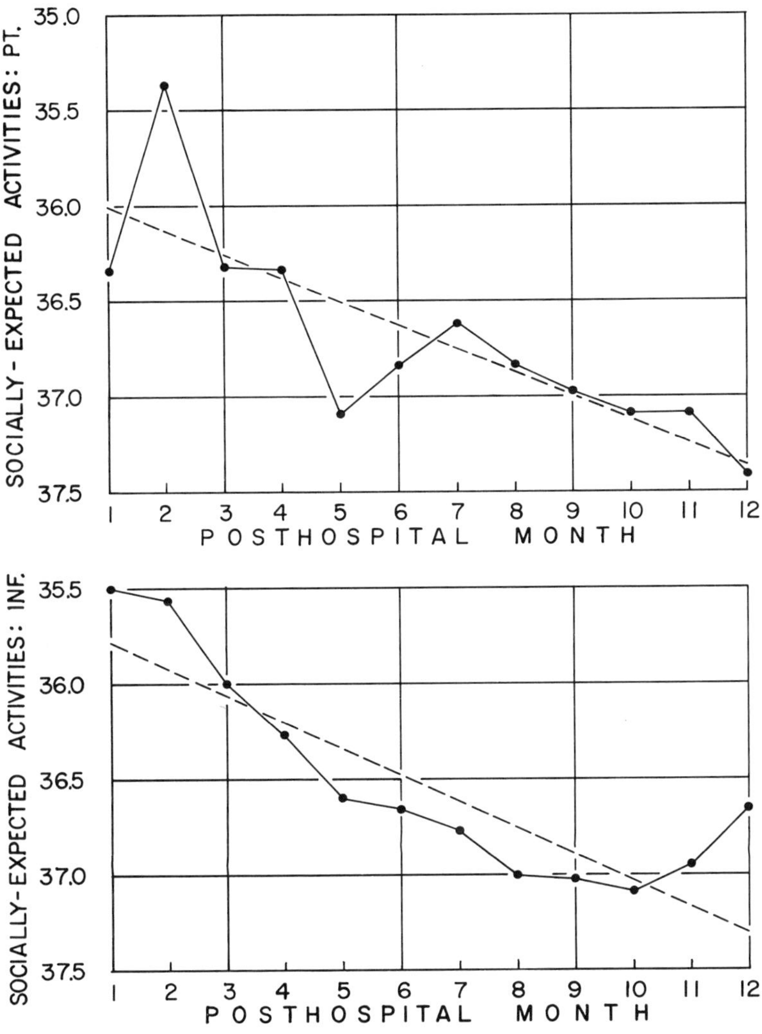


**Figure III-5. Monthly scores on KAS Socially-Expected Activities as reported by patients (top) and informants (bottom). Solid lines show mean raw scores of the complete nonrelapser group (*N* = 51). Broken lines show best-fit slopes: linear regression coefficient = .08 for patients, .09 for informants. On vertical axes, conventional high-low arrangement of scores is reversed so that downward direction means improvement, consistently with most of the other adjustment variables.**

among the three scales. Patients saw themselves as improving little if any in actual performance (*SEA-P*), but they had expected even less of themselves (*LOE-P*); hence their self-satisfaction (*SSA-P*),

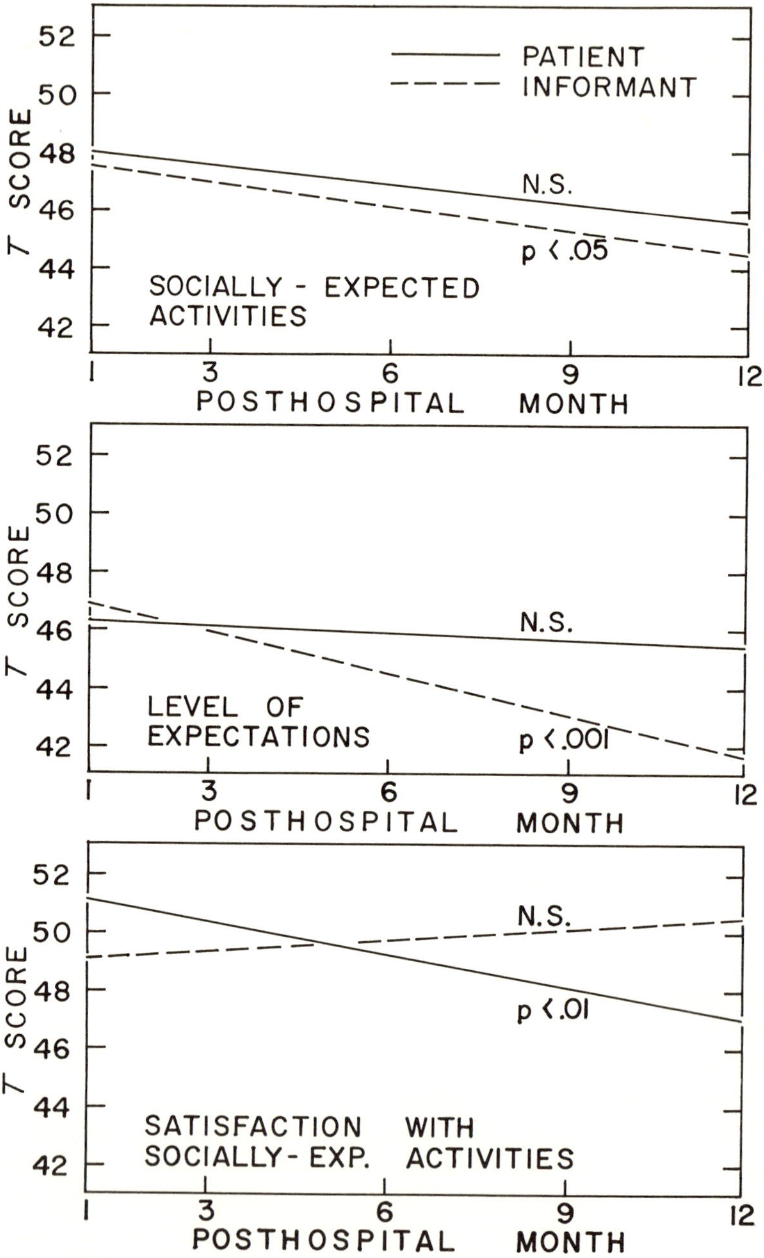


Figure III-6. Best-fit year-long trends for patient reports compared with informant reports on the three KAS measures pertaining to socially-expected activities. *T* scales are based on Month-1 scores of all participants ($N = 139$). To make high scores unfavorable throughout, raw-score directions are reversed in the top and middle graphs.

alone of the patient scales, improved significantly. With informants the month-to-month outlook was drastically different: their satisfaction with patients (*SSA-I*) was the only informant scale *not* registering improvement, and in fact they became nonsignificantly more disappointed as the year went by. Phenomenologically as well as psychometrically, their disappointment was predetermined by their having expected more of patients (*LOE-I*) than they saw them performing (*SEA-I*). Thus results again point up the need for counseling of patients' "significant others," aimed at realistically tempering their posthospital expectations. In a British posthospital study similar to our own, Wing, Monck, Brown, and Carstairs (1964) observed: "In the absence of effective community services, the policy of early discharge of schizophrenic patients is based to a large degree on [the] willingness of relatives to attempt the role of nurse and to put up with considerable discomfort and distress." Appropriately timed counseling of relatives, concerning tenable expectations for patients, could well constitute crisis prevention or crisis intervention in many cases.

## SUMMARY

Results presented in this chapter are those related most directly to the study's methodological innovations. It is hoped that our approaches can lead toward more effective models for outpatient treatment.

During the follow-up year, 52 (37.4 per cent) of the 139 participants were rehospitalized at least once, with a maximum of three readmissions for any patient. Participants averaged 46.6 days of additional inpatient time, while the 52 relapsers averaged 124.7 days with a range of 1 to 321. Monthly readmission rates showed no chronological "danger zones."

Most participants, and most relapsers as well, received outpatient treatment including chemotherapy at Month 1. Relapsers were for the most part still attending a clinic immediately before their first rehospitalization; however, drug treatment had been discontinued for a substantial number of these patients. For them, it seems possible that uninterrupted drug prescriptions would have averted rehospitalization in some if not all cases.

On each of the 26 adjustment variables, nonrelapsers were compared with relapsers at each of the 12 posthospital months; the in-community relapser group for these comparisons was of necessity reduced by sporadic rehospitalization, but was also augmented by those relapsers who returned to the community and resumed monthly testing. There were many significant monthly differences in adjustment, all favoring nonrelapsers. Informant-report measures discriminated relatively more often than patient-reported measures. In terms of manifest item content, "social" measures discriminated best, "psychopathological" measures next best, and "judgmental" measures least. Other data analyses showed that, taking into account initial adjustment at Month 1, relapsers ended the year with a less favorable "outcome" than nonrelapsers.

The 40 interview-based life-situation variables were less effective than the adjustment variables in registering monthly in-community differences between nonrelapsers and relapsers—perhaps partly because of methodological limitations. Work and homemaking was the life-situation area most sensitive to differences; here, as well as in the home-and-family area, nonrelapsers showed consistently greater social maturity. Neither patient nor informant life-situation reports proved superior as discriminators. In view of the combined results on adjustment and life situation in these longitudinal analyses, relapsers appear to have been following an inexorably and distinctively deteriorating course of adjustment, despite abundant outpatient and inpatient treatment.

At Month 1, in the total participants group, there were numerous meaningful concurrent relations between life-situation items and "global adjustment" as measured by a special KAS composite score. Close affiliation with parent(s) as opposed to spouse was especially associated with poor in-community adjustment, as was environmental stress via item-by-item analyses. The same analyses were made at Month 12 ($N = 94$), where significant relations between life-situation variables and global adjustment were fewer and presented a pattern different from that at Month 1. It was tentatively inferred that the very early posthospital period confronted patients with special social and environmental problems which to some extent they were able to master as the year progressed.

The 51 nonrelapsers who completed almost all of the 12 monthly tests provided opportunity for longitudinal study of a full uninterrupted year of in-community adjustment. Trend analyses indicated significant improvement on 16 variables and significant worsening on none. Test-retest effects, while probably present, did not appear to account entirely for the indicated improvement. Because of informants' unrealistically high expectations for patients' socially-expected activities, their disappointment with patients mounted throughout the posthospital year.

Chapter IV

# Predicting Adjustment

In contrast to Chapter III, most of the results presented here and in Chapter V resemble those of many conventionally designed posthospital studies—for example, the one by Freeman and Simmons (1963). Since elementary background variables were our only *pre-release* predictors of adjustment, however, we have less to offer for that particular kind of prediction than for predictions from early to later posthospital periods. In other words, few of our findings pertain to the problem of whom to discharge from the hospital, when, and how; most of them belong rather in the clinical context of aftercare planning and management: Who needs aftercare, and when? What are the prime target symptoms and critical danger signals? What should be done to minimize rehospitalizations?

The study design embodied three major sets of predictor variables which could be tested against some or all of three major adjustment criteria as indicated by "x":

| *Predictors* | *Criteria* | | |
|---|---|---|---|
| | Early posthospital adjustment | Late posthospital adjustment | Early-to-late outcome |
| Pre-release information | x | x | x |
| Early posthospital adjustment | | x | x |
| Early posthospital life situation | | x | x |

The terms "early" and "late" refer respectively to Months 1 and 12. Among the predictors, "pre-release information" consists of the background variables, seven demographic and five clinical; "posthospital adjustment" consists of the 26 adjustment variables; and "posthospital life situation" consists of the 40 life-situation variables. The "posthospital adjustment" criterion was the global adjustment score (Appendix O); the "early-to-late outcome" criterion was the outcome index (Figure III-3 and Appendix Q).[1]

## PREDICTING EARLY POSTHOSPITAL ADJUSTMENT

The relation between each background variable and Month-1 global adjustment was tested by $r$, $t$, or $F$ as appropriate. Three of the twelve predictors reached significance at or beyond the .025 level (Table IV-1, upper portion). All others failed to reach the .10 level. Paradigmatically, the patient with the worst prognosis for early posthospital adjustment is seen to have been a never-married schizophrenic with a comparatively long hospital stay during his only or most recent admission. Variables notably failing to predict early adjustment were age, sex, type of release, and the two indexes of prior hospitalization.

The marital status prediction parallels the relation already noted between type of home at Month 1 and concurrent global adjustment (Table III-9). Probably the most complex relation is that for length of last hospitalization. To suggest, on the basis of its low but significant negative correlation with good adjustment at

[1]When prediction is from early posthospital adjustment to either of its two indicated criteria, there is obvious predictor-criterion contamination. Primarily it is due to autocorrelation: The five KAS scores which are represented in each of the criteria are also among the 26 adjustment variables tested as predictors. (It will be seen, however that these five are not necessarily the most effective predictors.) Secondarily, contamination is aggravated to the extent that the same five KAS scores are correlated with the remaining 21 adjustment variables (Appendix M, Table M-1). In our opinion, this methodological objection is overridden by the potential usefulness of the implied clinical-practice prediction model (subject to cross-validation of our findings): a newly released patient's KAS profile can be used to forecast his later adjustment, and what is then being forecast is a score which approximates how that adjustment would be globally rated by clinicians after comprehensive interviews with the patient plus an informant. Or, if early-to-late *outcome* is to be forecast, the same elements are involved, in a more complex arrangement. In such situations, when treatment is being planned, prognostically favorable signs would constitute patient assets and unfavorable signs would point toward important target symptoms.

*Table IV-1. Background Variables Most Effectively Predicting Early and Late Global Adjustment*

| Variable | Global Adjustment Mean | Global Adjustment S.D. |
|---|---|---|
| Criterion: Month 1 ($N = 139$) | | |
| Marital status ($F = 5.37, p < .01$): | | |
| Single | 3.8* | 1.2 |
| Married | 4.6 | 1.2 |
| Widowed, separated, divorced | 3.9 | 1.5 |
| Mos. hospitalized last adm. ($r = -.23, p = .02$) | – | – |
| Diagnosis ($F = 3.80, p < .025$): | | |
| Schizophrenic reaction | 4.0* | 1.4 |
| Psychoses other than schizophrenia | 4.5 | 1.1 |
| Nonpsychotic disorders | 4.7 | 1.2 |
| Criterion: Month 12 ($N = 94$) | | |
| Years of education ($r = .24, p < .05$) | – | – |
| No. of prior hosp. ($r = -.22, p < .05$) | – | – |
| Type of release ($t = 1.69, p < .10$): | | |
| Convalescent leave | 4.5* | 1.3 |
| Discharge | 5.0 | 1.2 |

*Worst mean subgroup score for each variable.

Month 1, that we should always discharge patients as soon as possible, would be a gross misreading of the data. Rather, we are reminded again of Honigfeld and Gillis's (1967) finding of a pernicious positive relation, not dependent on patient age, between increasing length of hospitalization and increasing severity of schizophrenics' illness. Unquestionably those of our patients who had the longer hospitalizations were generally those who needed them; yet here again our data intimate that treatment may at best have only been containing the illness and providing temporary environmental surcease for patients and/or their affiliates. It was not the longest-treated patients who emerged best-adjusted.

## PREDICTING LATE POSTHOSPITAL ADJUSTMENT

In testing predictions involving Month-12 evaluations we were limited to the 94 patients in the previously described anchor-months cohort, i.e., those who completed not only Test 1 but also Test 12, and for whom Test 12 was not a relapse test. Clinically, a member of this group was a patient who may or may not have been rehospitalized during the year but who, if he did re-enter a hospital, was back in the community at Month 12 and thereby available for testing at that time.

*Adjustment Predicted from Background Variables*

In predicting Month-12 global adjustment we again begin with, but are here not limited to, background variables (Table IV-1, lower portion). Again there were three comparatively successful predictors, but in no instance did the same background variable predict adjustment at both anchor months.[2] On the other hand, the clinical background variables as a class were prepotently successful at both months, with two out of five significant at each month as opposed to only one out of seven demographic background variables likewise effective at each month. The typical poorly adjusted patient at Month 12 had little education and one or more prior hospitalizations; he had left the hospital on convalescent leave, not direct discharge.

The mean global adjustment of 3.8 for never-married patients at Month 1 is the worst found among the subgroup discriminations in Table IV-1. In the calibration of this scale (Appendix O) it represents a point very close to what clinical raters consider "about average for ex-hospitalized patients"–viz., 4.0. The best average adjustment was that of 5.0 at Month 12 for patients on direct discharge; on the global adjustment scale the clinician rates a patient 5 if he considers that his "overall functioning is above average for ex-hospitalized patients," but not near the upper limit of good adjustment.

*Adjustment Predicted from Adjustment Variables*

To test the relation of each Month-1 adjustment score to Month-12 global adjustment, Pearson *r*s were computed. Table IV-2 presents complete results, including the few variables that did not attain the .05 significance level. Nineteen of the 26 Month-1

[2]Diagnosis, however, yielded an $F$ ratio of 1.70, $p < .20$, in the Month-12 analysis. Mean global-adjustment scores for the three diagnostic groups were in the same rank order as at Month 1 (Table IV-1).

*Table IV-2. Early Adjustment Scores as Predictors of Late Global Adjustment*

| Variable | *r* | *p* .01 | *p* .02 or .05 | *p* .10 or N.S. |
|---|---|---|---|---|
| KAS–Patient only: | | | | |
| *Sym* | –.10 | | | N.S. |
| KAS–Patient (see also Informant below): | | | | |
| *SEA-P* | .35[a] | .01 | | |
| *LOE-P* | .38[a] | .01 | | |
| *SSA-P* | –.12 | | | N.S. |
| *FTA-P* | –.13 | | | N.S. |
| *SFA-P* | –.11 | | | N.S. |
| KAS–Informant only: | | | | |
| *Bel* | –.37 | .01 | | |
| *Exp* | –.27 | .01 | | |
| *Neg* | –.31 | .01 | | |
| *Hel* | –.25 | | .02 | |
| *Sus* | –.41 | .01 | | |
| *Anx* | –.23 | | .05 | |
| *Wdl* | –.24 | | .02 | |
| *Psy* | –.45 | .01 | | |
| *Ner* | –.38 | .01 | | |
| *Con* | –.18 | | | .10 |
| *Biz* | –.28 | .01 | | |
| *Hyp* | –.21 | | .05 | |
| *Sta* | .26[a] | .01 | | |
| KAS–Informant (see also Patient above): | | | | |
| *SEA-I* | .38[a] | .01 | | |
| *LOE-I* | .21[a] | | .05 | |
| *SSA-I* | –.31 | .01 | | |
| *FTA-I* | –.20 | | .05 | |
| *SFA-I* | –.31 | .01 | | |
| Stress Index: | | | | |
| *Str-P* | .02 | | | N.S. |
| *Str-I* | .00 | | | N.S. |

[a]For these five variables only, positive *r* values indicate that favorable early adjustment is associated with favorable late adjustment and conversely. For all other variables, *r* must be negative to indicate the same correspondence.

adjustment scores did significantly predict end-of-year global adjustment, and 13 of the 19 were highly significant ($p < .01$).

Relations were always in the expected direction except for the stress indexes, both of which had zero-order correlations: The effects of Month-1 environmental stress are not registered at Month 12. We have noted earlier the apparently special impact of early posthospital stress on the patient and the possibility of his gradual adaptation to stress throughout the year. The present findings also support that outlook. So does the fact that correlations between stress and adjustment scores are generally higher at Month 1 than at Month 12 (Appendix M, Table M-2, rows 4a-5b)—although the correlation differences are probably related to the test-retest phenomena described by Howard (1964).

Informants were decisively better "predictors" than patients: Except for *Str-I* (Informant Stress), only one of their 19 scales failed to reach the .05 level—*Con* (Confusion). As to manifest content of the scales, all three categories (psychopathological, social, judgmental) were adequately represented among the effective predictor variables. However, neither of the two patient-reported psychopathological scales predicted successfully. In fact, the only two successful patient scales, *SEA* (Performance of Socially-Expected Activities) and *LOE* (Level of Expectations), were those embodied in the global adjustment criterion (footnote 1 above; Appendix O). Consistently with other results (Table III-6), clinically meaningful discriminations among patients are better accomplished via informants than by the patients themselves. Despite informants' general superiority in this respect, however, Table IV-2 indicates that patients' reports on *LOE* predicted somewhat more accurately than did informants'. But this was not the case with the indirect measure of satisfaction, *SSA* (Satisfaction with Socially-Expected Activities), where the informants' predictive superiority was markedly evident.

Considered singly, the two best predictors were the psychopathological scales *Psy* (General Psychopathology) and *Sus* (Suspiciousness), with *r*s of -.45 and -.41. Also of interest is a question not covered in Table IV-2: To what extent does the criterion measure predict itself? The correlation between Month-1 and Month-12 global adjustment was .43, $p < .01$.

### *Adjustment Predicted from Life-Situation Variables*

The *F* test (one-way analysis of variance) was used to determine relations between life situation at Month 1 and global adjustment at Month 12. Expectedly, useful results were considerably fewer here than among adjustment variables. None of the 40 life-situation variables at Month 1 predicted late posthospital adjustment at the .05 level; only 14 yielded $F$ ratios as large as 1.0. Of these, the eight most nearly reaching significance are shown in Table IV-3. This is another set of findings which could be dismissed as perhaps essentially random, except that for the most part the pattern makes sense clinically and accords with results of other analyses.

The risk of inferior adjustment at Month 12 was greatest for patients whose closest affiliation was non-conjugal, especially if it was parental; who were relatively unproductive as wage-earners; and who *were* involved in aftercare. Prediction results were in the hypothesized direction only for one of the two tabulated stress items, economic and domestic. Patients who reported *no* marital-sexual stress at Month 1 were in worse condition at Month 12 than those who did report stress in that area. We shall defer comment on this paradox until we consider its reappearance in predictions of early-to-late outcome (Table IV-6).

Patient and informant as sources of data were once again about equally represented in their proportionate shares of the most nearly significant life-situation discriminators. Among life-situation areas, there was some imbalance: work and homemaking again carried greatest discriminative weight, home and family was fairly represented, and treatment as well as stress contributed less than their expected share.

## PREDICTING END-OF-YEAR OUTCOME

Predictions of adjustment status at a certain point in time, such as those just presented, are often sought by administrators and public health statisticians. Of greater relevance for the clinician, in the daily decisions he must make in accepting and treating patients, are predictions of *outcome*. To help a patient optimally, he must know which aspects of his current condition and circumstances are premonitory and which are auspicious—not generally, but *given* the patient's own presenting condition as a starting point for therapeutic effort, and with improvement as a goal of treat-

*Table IV-3. Early Life Situation Variables Most Effectively Predicting Late Global Adjustment*

| Life Situation | | Global Adjustment | |
|---|---|---|---|
| Item | Respondent, N | Mean | S.D. |
| Home and Family | | | |
| Closest living relative ($p < .10$): | Patient | | |
| Spouse | 74 | 4.8 | 1.2 |
| Parent, child, or sibling | 20 | 4.1* | 1.3 |
| Informant ($p < .20$): | Informant | | |
| Spouse | 50 | 4.8 | 1.2 |
| Parent | 16 | 4.0* | 1.3 |
| Son or daughter | 10 | 5.0 | 0.7 |
| Sibling | 9 | 4.9 | 1.3 |
| All other | 9 | 4.2 | 1.5 |
| Work and Homemaking | | | |
| Busiest single work week ($p < .20$):[a] | Patient | | |
| Less than full time | 5 | 4.2* | 1.3 |
| Full time or more | 15 | 5.3 | 1.1 |
| Busiest single work week ($p < .20$):[a] | Informant | | |
| Less than full time | 4 | 4.2* | 1.5 |
| Full time or more | 15 | 5.3 | 1.2 |
| Breadwinner contribution ($p < .20$):[a] | Informant | | |
| No contribution | 57 | 4.5* | 1.3 |
| Less than major | 18 | 4.9 | 1.2 |
| Sole or major breadwinner | 10 | 5.2 | 1.2 |
| Treatment | | | |
| Outlook for future ($p < .10$): | Patient | | |
| No plan to continue or start | 22 | 5.1 | 1.3 |
| Plan to continue or start | 72 | 4.5* | 1.2 |
| Stress | | | |
| Marital and sexual stress ($p < .10$): | Patient | | |
| Some | 21 | 5.1 | 1.0 |
| None | 73 | 4.5* | 1.3 |
| Economic and domestic stress ($p < .20$): | Patient | | |
| Some | 33 | 4.4* | 1.2 |
| None | 61 | 4.8 | 1.3 |

*Worst mean subgroup score for each variable.

[a]Some cases excluded; see Appendix R.

ment. This kind of consideration is central to our analyses of outcome predictions, based on the same anchor-months cohort

($N$ = 94) as in the above predictions of late posthospital adjustment. The criterion was dichotomous as shown previously in Figure III-3: Favorable outcome ($N$ = 53) *vs.* unfavorable outcome ($N$ = 41).

*Outcome Predicted from Background Variables*

Relations with outcome were tested by chi square for nonparametric background variables and by $t$ for parametric background variables. As it happened, significant results were found only among the latter (Table IV-4). None of the remaining eight background variables attained a predictive significance level better than $p < .50$–including age, sex, marital status, education, diagnosis, and type of release. In Table IV-4, poor posthospital prognosis is indicated for patients with fewer children, greater prior hospitalization experience, and longer confinement during most recent or only admission. Clinical background variables as a group predicted more effectively than demographic variables.

*Table IV-4. Background Variables Most Effectively Predicting Outcome*

| Variable | Outcome | | | |
|---|---|---|---|---|
| | Favorable | | Unfavorable | |
| | Mean | S.D. | Mean | S.D. |
| No. of children ($p < .05$) | 2.3 | 1.8 | 1.8 | 1.4 |
| No. of prior hosp. ($p < .01$) | 1.8 | 2.2 | 2.8 | 2.8 |
| Years of prior hosp. ($p < .10$) | 0.9 | 2.0 | 1.6 | 3.2 |
| Mos. hospitalized last adm. ($p < .01$) | 3.2 | 3.8 | 5.2 | 11.5 |

*Note:* All $p$ values based on $t$, two-tailed test.

It is not clear why number of children was the only significant demographic variable. The reason may have to do with this variable's dual psychosocial implications: Children represent not only past achievement in living but also a compelling inducement to constructive posthospital functioning. The remaining three predictors all connote adverse effects of hospitalization experience. Viewed in conjunction with the nonsignificant relation of age to outcome ($p < .90$), they bear out the previously cited findings of Honigfeld and Gillis (1967) and the authors' recommendation: "In order to maximize the natural, health-directed propensities of the organism, every effort should be made to avoid prolonged institutionalization."

In a sample of 100 female inpatients descriptively similar to our own subjects, Barry and Fulkerson (1966) found that, contrary to expectations, "*poor* [cognitive and psychomotor] test performance among acute patients is associated with a shorter stay in the [private] hospital." Their acute patients were those with comparatively recent onset of illness. In our own study, by using "education" in place of test scores and by defining "acute" as "no prior hospitalizations," we were able to investigate a similar interaction in the 30 first-admission patients in the anchor-months cohort, with reference not to in-hospital experience but to posthospital outcome. Education was dichotomized at the median, 10.8 years. Results ($p < .10$) were consonant with those of Barry and Fulkerson, as 60 per cent of the 20 acute patients whose outcome was favorable were in the low-education group, while 80 per cent of the 10 with unfavorable outcome had high education. Moreover, a converse tendency ($p < .20$) was found in our 64 "chronics" (patients with at least one prior hospitalization): under favorable outcome ($N$ = 33), 58 per cent had high education, while under unfavorable outcome ($N$ = 31) 61 per cent had low education. We have no ready explanation for this finding that education tended to be a therapeutic liability for our acute patients and an asset for chronics; the issue merits further study by other investigators.

*Outcome Predicted from Adjustment Variables*

Seven of the 26 Month-1 adjustment measures predicted outcome at significance levels from .01 to .10 (Table IV-5). Five of these were correlated with the outcome index at the .05 level—viz., the first four variables tabulated, plus *Bel* (Belligerence), which had an $r$ of -.27, $p < .01$, but failed to predict the dichotomous criterion ($p < .50$) and therefore does not appear in the table.

At Month 1, considering first only the psychopathological variables, patients whose outcome was to be comparatively unsuccessful were generally those whose informants described them as excessively suspicious, inordinately afflicted with a variety of heterogeneous symptoms, and lacking in emotional stability. None

*Table IV-5. Early Adjustment Variables Most Effectively Predicting Outcome*

| Variable | $p^a$ | Favorable Outcome | | Unfavorable Outcome | | $r^b$ |
|---|---|---|---|---|---|---|
| | | Mean | S.D. | Mean | S.D. | |
| *KAS*–Patient: | | | | | | |
| *LOE-P*[c] | .05 | 37.3 | 4.9 | 35.1 | 4.7 | .23 |
| *SSA-P* | .10 | 9.2 | 8.9 | 6.1 | 7.3 | .23 |
| *KAS*–Informant: | | | | | | |
| *Sus* | .05 | 4.9 | 1.7 | 5.8 | 2.3 | –.24 |
| *Psy* | .10 | 33.9 | 7.6 | 37.4 | 9.6 | –.23 |
| *Sta*[c] | .10 | 30.1 | 5.1 | 28.2 | 5.5 | .05 |
| *SSA-I* | .01 | 4.3 | 5.4 | 8.0 | 7.8 | –.17 |
| *SFA-I* | .05 | 29.0 | 4.8 | 31.2 | 5.5 | –.16 |

[a]Based on two-tailed *t*-tests of differences between the tabulated means.

[b]Early adjustment variable correlated with outcome index; *p* values not tabulated.

[c]On these two adjustment variables only, high scores are favorable. Results must be interpreted accordingly.

of these results is surprising; the psychopathological variables were neither under- nor overrepresented among the sensitive outcome predictors. Social variables were entirely absent, though they proved effective in other analyses. So were the two stress indexes–an indication that, while stress did figure in adjustment at certain junctures, its presence at Month 1 did not cast a long shadow.

It was the judgmental variables which were most informative in outcome predictions, both proportionately and qualitatively. *LOE-P* results showed that high Month-1 goals for one's own social performance augured well for outcome and vice versa. Most striking in this area was the divergence of patient and informant discriminations on *SSA*. Patients in the favorable outcome group were comparatively *dissatisfied* with their own Month-1 social performance, while for the same individuals their onlookers reported themselves to have been relatively *satisfied.* For the patients themselves the dynamics seem similar to those found in psychotherapeutic practice and research. For informants, it appears that whatever their Month-1 attitudes had to do with outcome was more akin to nurturance or supportiveness than to coaching or coaxing. The lack of predictive discrimination via direct reports of social performance itself, from both respondents, highlights the intrapsychic process involved in *SSA-P* (Satisfaction with Socially-Expected Activities–Patient) and the transactional importance of *SSA-I*. (It will be remembered that many informants were spouses.)

In Table IV-5 as a whole, patients and informants each had roughly their fair share of discriminators. Only two other adjustment variables (not listed) showed predictive power approaching that of those we have examined: *Anx* (Anxiety) ($p < .30$) and *Ner* (Nervousness) ($p < .20$). On both, the favorable outcome group had the better mean scores at Month 1.

*Outcome Predicted from Life-Situation Variables*[3]

It is clear from Table IV-6 that life situation was generally a statistically negligible area as regards prediction of outcome. Only five variables reached a significance level of .20 or better; none of these was in the work and homemaking area and only one was a treatment variable. Despite these meager results, some of the predictions compel attention within the perspective of emerging results from several analyses.

We have shown that the backgound variable "number of children" predicted outcome (Table IV-4) and have conjectured as to its special power in this regard. That finding is reinforced by the fact that outcome also depended on how many children were living at home with the patient–a number often smaller than the total child count.

In the treatment area, the only predictor approaching significance was "outlook for future." This variable, an index of present plus anticipated involvement, has now discriminated recurrently and consistently thoughout several major analyses, always in the direction of earmarking treated patients as sicker (Tables III-8, III-9, III-10, IV-3, IV-6). If treatment had distinctly benefitted recipients throughout the year, such results would hardly have been likely. On the other hand, many of the treated patients, had they been without such help, might well have moved through the year in worse condition than was actually the case. Further con-

[3]Under this heading, two life-situation variables were untestable because of skewed distributions: (1) Step-, in-law children in home, and (2) social and recreational stress (informant's report).

*Table IV-6. Early Life Situation Variables Most Effectively Predicting Outcome*

| Item | Outcome: Favorable *N* | Favorable Per Cent | Unfavorable *N* | Unfavorable Per Cent |
|---|---|---|---|---|
| Home and Family | | | | |
| Own children in home (Pt.,[a] $p < .05$): | | | | |
| None | 18 | 34 | 25 | 61 |
| One | 16 | 30 | 7 | 17 |
| Two to six | 19 | 36 | 9 | 22 |
| Closest living relative (Pt., $p < .10$): | | | | |
| Spouse | 46 | 87 | 28 | 68 |
| All other | 7 | 13 | 13 | 32 |
| Treatment | | | | |
| Outlook for future (Pt., $p < .20$): | | | | |
| No plan to continue or start | 16 | 30 | 6 | 15 |
| Plan to continue or start | 37 | 70 | 35 | 85 |
| Stress | | | | |
| "Bad" event(s) during month (Inf.,[a] $p < .20$): | | | | |
| One or more | 19 | 36 | 21 | 51 |
| None | 34 | 64 | 20 | 49 |
| Marital and sexual stress (Pt., $p < .10$): | | | | |
| Some | 16 | 30 | 5 | 12 |
| None | 37 | 70 | 36 | 88 |

[a]Respondent: Pt. (patient), Inf. (informant).

trolled studies designed to resolve such speculations are much to be desired.

Marital and sexual stress (reported almost always in the marital context) is an item which has sometimes confirmed, at other times disconfirmed, our hypothesis regarding stress as an antitherapeutic force.[4] Obviously, the area is one of intense, enduring, and telling transactional ferment; even in our testing sessions some patient-informant couples were observably allied in love and solicitude while others were openly antagonistic to the point of disparagement and ridicule. Marital stress unquestionably deserves additional and closer study in the elucidation of posthospital adjustment. We suspect that the key to the paradoxically beneficial correlates of marital stress is contained in Jerome D. Frank's pos-

[4]A third confirmation is reported in Chapter V.

tulate concerning emotional arousal as a common denominator of many effective "influencing processes" including psychotherapy. As paraphrased by Yahraes (1967, p. 213), Frank's outlook is that: "Basic to the success of all these processes . . . is a state of emotional tension or arousal, however this is reached. Generally involved, too, is an influencing agent, who acts as a stimulator of emotion, a model with whom the attitude changer can identify, and a source of new information and logical argument. . . . The researcher also believes that a change in one attitude, no matter by what influencing process it is accomplished, generally leads to changes in other attitudes."

## SUMMARY

Three sets of variables were tested as predictors of posthospital adjustment: pre-release information (background variables), early posthospital adjustment (Month-1 adjustment scores), and early posthospital life situation (Month-1 life-situation reports). Three criteria of adjustment were all based on the KAS global adjustment score: early posthospital adjustment (Month 1), late posthospital adjustment (Month 12), and early-to-late outcome (a refined change score or outcome index based on initial and final scores). Only background variables were available as testable predictors of Month-1 global adjustment. Patients with poor adjustment at Month 1 were typically never-married schizophrenics with comparatively long recent hospitalizations.

In predictions of Month-12 global adjustment, the poorest prognosis in terms of background variables was indicated for convalescent-leave patients with low education and one or more prior hospitalizations. Among numerous Month-1 adjustment scores showing poor risk for Month 12, the most potent predictors were the KAS informant scales *Psy* and *Sus*. Month-1 life-situation variables were much less effective than adjustment variables in forecasting end-of-year adjustment.

Patients with a poor end-of-year outcome were those with fewer children and more inpatient experience. On the Month-1 KAS they were deviant in some aspects of symptomatology, expectations, and satisfaction, but not in social behavior. Life-situation variables again were comparatively ineffective as prognostic indicators.

When the results of the various analyses are cross-checked with each other, a number of sensitive issues are discernible. Their implications are stated as they bear upon the posthospital adjustment process, the role of treatment in the patient's changing condition, and the need for further investigation of certain questions.

Chapter V

# Predicting Rehospitalization

This chapter will show that, at the end of the first posthospital month, it may be possible for aftercare clinicians to identify relapse-prone patients accurately enough to warrant devoting special therapeutic attention to them. Indications for suitable treatment approaches with such cases are also developed. The forecasting of readmission *vs.* staying out of the hospital depends, as will be seen, on predictor variables representing all three of our data categories: background, adjustment, and life situation.

Numerous studies of rehospitalization are to be found in the literature. In addition to those we have cited, the problem is dealt with in reports by Johnston and McNeal (1965); Lorei (1964); Schooler, Goldberg, Boothe, and Cole (1967); Sherman, Moseley, Ging, and Bookbinder (1964); and Vaillant (1964). Our own work on rehospitalization differs in three ways from most of these. First, as in Chapter IV, predictors consist largely of early *post*-discharge measures and hence have little to do with guidelines for discharge decisions. Second, our longitudinal repeated-measurements method enables us to study rehospitalization in relation not only to the patient's status at given points earlier in time, but also in relation to the entire course of his posthospital adjustment, up to the moment of readmission. Third, we examine in considerable detail the patient's environmental stress as a condition antecedent to rehospitalization.

For predictions in this chapter, the criterion was the simple dichotomy of no rehospitalization during the follow-up year (nonrelapser) *vs.* one or more rehospitalizations (relapser). Let us restate several points on the limitations of this criterion: It is essentially practical and phenomenological, and it leaves much to be desired both methodologically and heuristically, despite its formidable clinical significance. (For example, one of our nonrelapsers was rehospitalized on the next day after she finished her study year.) Moreover, the rehospitalization criterion is subject to three logistical limitations peculiar to this study: (1) noninclusion of patients who relapsed within the first 20 days; (2) sampling bias with relapsers somewhat overrepresented and vice versa; and (3) the possibility that a very few incompletes were erroneously classified as nonrelapsers by our failure to detect their rehospitalization at other institutions.

## PREDICTION FROM BACKGROUND VARIABLES

### *Univariate Predictions*

Six of the 12 background variables showed virtually no predictive relations to rehospitalization: $p$ values ranged from .50 to .80. Five of these were demographic: Age, sex, number of children, religion, and occupation. The one least effective clinical variable was "months hospitalized during last admission."

Tables V-I and V-2 present the variables which reached or most nearly approached significance. They are based on the entire participant sample comprising 87 nonrelapsers and 52 relapsers. The patient with greatest risk of rehospitalization was the poorly educated, often hospitalized schizophrenic who left Spring Grove on convalescent leave. Total duration of prior hospitalizations also contributed positively to relapse risk, as did nonmarried status to a slight degree. Clinical background variables as a group were better predictors than demographic items, here as in our previous major prediction tests.

Of special interest are the results for the three variables pertaining to inpatient experience. There is no evidence that some patients may have been prematurely discharged just before starting the study, since duration of last hospitalization did not predict

*Table V-1. Nonparametric Background Variables Most Effectively Predicting Rehospitalization*

| Variable | Nonrelapsers | | Relapsers | |
|---|---|---|---|---|
| | $N$ | Per Cent | $N$ | Per Cent |
| Demographic | | | | |
| Marital status ($p < .25$): | | | | |
| Single | 12 | 14 | 12 | 23 |
| Married | 59 | 68 | 28 | 54 |
| Widowed, separated, divorced | 16 | 18 | 12 | 23 |
| Clinical | | | | |
| Diagnosis ($p < .025$): | | | | |
| Schizophrenic reaction | 40 | 46 | 36 | 69 |
| Psychoses other than schizophrenia | 22 | 25 | 6 | 12 |
| Nonpsychotic disorders | 25 | 29 | 10 | 19 |
| Type of release ($p < .10$): | | | | |
| Convalescent leave | 68 | 78 | 47 | 90 |
| Discharge | 19 | 22 | 5 | 10 |

*Table V-2. Parametric Background Variables Most Effectively Predicting Rehospitalization*

| Variable | Nonrelapsers | | Relapsers | |
|---|---|---|---|---|
| | Mean | S.D. | Mean | S.D. |
| Demographic | | | | |
| Years of education ($p < .10$) | 10.8 | 3.0 | 9.9 | 2.4 |
| Clinical | | | | |
| No. of prior hosp. ($p < .001$) | 1.8 | 2.2 | 3.4 | 2.8 |
| Yrs. hosp. before last adm. ($p < .10$) | 1.0 | 2.4 | 1.9 | 2.6 |

*Note:* All $p$ values based on $t$, two-tailed test. For "years hospitalized before last admission" there were seven "unknown" cases which reduced the $N$s to 82 nonrelapsers and 50 relapsers.

relapse. But both variables dealing with amount of *prior* hospitalization were related to *subsequent* hospitalization, with total number of prior admissions being the most effective of all background predictors. The dictum that past behavior is the best predictor of future behavior, familiar in education and penology, seems to hold here. In fact, number of prior hospitalizations now stands as the most consistently powerful background variable in our whole series of prediction analyses. It also proved differentially sensitive in a controlled study of outpatient chemotherapy by Engelhardt, Freedman, and Mann (1963), which included some never-hospitalized subjects. We would therefore stress the importance of this variable as regards future investigations of outpatient treatment and adjustment. Our findings on the age variable, here and elsewhere, prove that it was not a predetermining factor in predictions based on prior hospitalization.

Four background variables have now yielded consistently negative results in the major prognostic analyses for adjustment and rehospitalization: age, sex, religion, and occupation. Two others have predicted both of these criteria only at borderline significance levels: years hospitalized before last admission, and type of release. Successful predictors of both criteria, at the .05 level or better, are number of hospitalizations prior to last, and diagnosis. The remaining four background variables did not significantly predict rehospitalization, but did predict one or more aspects of adjustment: marital status, number of children, education, and months hospitalized last admission.

By using data originally collected to evaluate sampling bias (Appendix N), we were able in a limited subsample to test one other descriptive variable as a predictor of rehospitalization. That variable was the distance in air miles from the patient's home to Spring Grove; the information was available on 26 nonrelapsers and 17 relapsers, but did not discriminate between them by $t$ test ($p < .40$), though relapsers did live on the average about two-and-one-half miles closer to the hospital than nonrelapsers.[1]

### *Interactions among Predictors*

When sex was controlled, diagnosis predicted rehospitalization more efficiently for females ($p < .01$) than for all participants, but failed to predict for males ($p < .90$). Among females, schizophrenics were ultra-prone to relapse, while patients with other psychoses and nonpsychotic diagnoses were more apt to avoid readmission.

[1]Among nonparticipants, essentially the same results were found when comparing 21 nonrelapsers with 13 relapsers.

When diagnosis was controlled, however, sex still failed as a predictor, although in the schizophrenic group females showed a slight tendency toward higher relapse rates than males ($p < .20$) .

No significant interaction was found between sex and marital status, regardless of which variable was controlled.

In Chapter IV we reported a paradoxically patterned interaction tendency between education and number of prior hospitalizations in the prediction of adjustment outcome, with low education auguring favorably for first-admission patients and vice versa. We investigated the same interaction with reference to the prediction of rehospitalization—controlling for number of prior hospitalizations and predicting from education dichotomized. With this criterion there were no such differential tendencies for education.

## PREDICTION FROM EARLY ADJUSTMENT VARIABLES

When returning home after psychiatric hospitalization, a patient undergoes drastic shifts of environment and social role. There is evidence that such changes, whether desirable or undesirable for the individual, are antecedently associated with physical and psychiatric illness (Rahe, McKean, and Arthur, 1967; Michaux, 1959). To the returning mental patient the home situation is not an unfamiliar one; yet vital continuities have been broken and must immediately be recommenced—with family, neighbors, friends, and perhaps employer. Our Month-1 measures of adjustment and life situation, here analyzed as predictors of rehospitalization, reflect the first 30 days of this effort to reconstitute the personal world. Clearly, this pivotal period could be a crucial one for subsequent avoidance or occurrence of rehospitalization.

More generally, certain aspects of admission procedures in Maryland point up the need for investigating related psychosocial processes. During the first year of our study, state mental hygiene officials reported that "the individual and his family are increasingly becoming the focal point in the decision to enter the [Maryland] mental hospital for treatment" (Tuerk and Gorwitz, 1963b). Voluntary admissions and admissions by relative's request had recently increased markedly and were together accounting for more than half of all hospitalizations of patients in our diagnostic groups, with relatives' requests in the majority. In this connection, the relevance of our data on how patients saw themselves and how they were seen by informants (most of whom were close relatives) is self-evident.

Four of our 52 relapsers returned to the hospital so early that their Month-1 test was a relapse test, i.e., it was taken after, not before, rehospitalization. We therefore removed these cases from the Month-1 prediction analyses of adjustment and of life situation, leaving 48 relapsers plus the intact group of 87 nonrelapsers. Tables V-3 and V-4 are based on these two groups.

*Main Results*

At Month 1, relapsers had worse average scores than nonrelapsers on 23 of the 26 adjustment variables. The three exceptions (all with *t*-test *p* values from .70 to .90) were *Sym* (Symptom Discomfort), *Str-P* (Patient Stress), and *Str-I* (Informant Stress). Six adjustment variables discriminated between nonrelapsers and relapsers at or well beyond the .10 level (Table V-3).[2] Grossly, the

*Table V-3. Early Adjustment Variables Most Effectively Predicting Rehospitalization*

| Variable | $p^a$ | Nonrelapsers | | Relapsers | |
|---|---|---|---|---|---|
| | | Mean | S.D. | Mean | S.D. |
| KAS–Patient: | | | | | |
| *SEA-P*[b] | .01 | 35.9 | 5.2 | 33.2 | 5.4 |
| *SSA-P* | .01 | 6.4 | 7.2 | 10.7 | 9.7 |
| KAS–Informant: | | | | | |
| *Psy* | .05 | 34.4 | 8.6 | 37.9 | 10.1 |
| *SEA-I*[b] | .10 | 35.3 | 5.1 | 33.5 | 4.7 |
| *SSA-I* | .05 | 5.1 | 6.0 | 7.8 | 7.4 |
| *SFA-I* | .001 | 28.9 | 4.8 | 33.0 | 5.9 |

[a]Based on two-tailed *t*-tests of differences between the tabulated means.

[b]On these two adjustment variables only, high scores are favorable. Results must be interpreted accordingly.

[2]Additionally, differences on six variables, all from the informant's KAS, were significant at $p < .20$: *Sus* (Suspiciousness), *Wdl* (Withdrawal and Retardation), *Con* (Confusion), *Biz* (Bizarreness), *Sta* (Emotional Stability), and *FTA-I* (Free-Time Activities–Informant).

relapsers thus appear to have been disadvantaged in adjustment as early as Month 1. Although specific interpretations are risky without cross-validation, the over-all results show that efforts to prevent rehospitalization would do well to begin with patients who manifest relatively poor adjustment during their first few posthospital weeks, even though relapse may not be imminent at that time. Compositely, the relapse-prone patient is characterized more by low social effectiveness than by any pattern of specific symptoms. Neither he nor his informant is satisfied with his social behavior; and the informant is particularly discontented with the way the patient spends his free time.

Table V-3 indicates that, as in predicting outcome, useful information would be lost by relying on either respondent to the exclusion of the other. While *SEA* (Performance of Socially-Expected Activities) and *SSA* (Satisfaction with Socially-Expected Activities) were effective predictors for both respondents and while no other patient-reported variables were effective, only *SEA* shows appreciable inter-respondent agreement at Month 1 (Appendix M, Table M-1); patients and informants did not agree closely in their level of satisfaction with patients' social performance, yet both of these matching satisfaction measures differentiated nonrelapsers from relapsers.

In content, the two *SSA* measures are judgmental. In the same category is *SFA-I* (Satisfaction with Free-Time Activities–Informant). Thus judgmental variables were relatively more successful predictively than either the fairly successful social variables–*SEA*, patient and informant–or the psychopathological category, here represented only by *Psy* (General Psychopathology). Patients destined to be rehospitalized were not, in the main, those who were decidedly sicker at Month 1, but those whose ordinary behavior simply engendered less *satisfaction* both in themselves and in their close affiliates. This predictive pattern is particularly meaningful in the light of patients' and relatives' often crucial roles in hospital decisions.

### *The Adjustment Variables in Retrospect*

Four adjustment variables have now proved surpassingly sensitive throughout the major analyses of course of adjustment

(Tables III-6, III-7, III-13), prediction of adjustment (Tables IV-2, IV-5), and prediction of rehospitalization (Table V-3)—yielding one or more results significant at or beyond the .05 level in each area. They are the patient social variable *SEA*, the informant psychopathological variable *Psy*, and the informant judgmental variables *SSA* and *SFA*. If one had to choose the adjustment variables of greatest clinical import in aftercare, on the basis of our composite results, he would surely begin with these four. Closely following these as choices on the same basis would be the patient judgmental variable *SSA* and the informant social variable *SEA*. The few most sensitive variables are heterogeneous as regards both respondent and content area; for complete clinical or investigative data coverage, then, one cannot afford to completely exclude the patient, the informant, or any of the three content categories.

The reader will recall that the satisfaction measure *SSA* is based on the discrepancy between performance (*SEA*) and expectations (*LOE*) (Level of Expectations). What is striking about this triad in Table V-3 is that relapse is not predicted by the early *expectations* of either informant, but is predicted by both respondents' reports of social *performance, and* by the *discrepancy* between expectations and performance, again with both respondents represented. Our data have already shown that relatives may need counseling against inordinately high expectations (Figure II-1). Indirectly, Table V-3 reiterates that implication and shows further that patients could often benefit from similar advice. It is easy to envision the kind of discontent that *SSA* measures, in both parties, as being dynamically crucial in those interpersonal processes which culminate in rehospitalization. A South African field study by Gillis and Keet (1965) vividly documents the transactional power of "the attitudes and actions of the family, and particularly of the significant relative," in hospitalizations of schizophrenic patients. Lorei (1964) demonstrated that relatives' attitudes as measured by questionnaire were related to length of stay out of the hospital.

The other satisfaction measure, *SFA*, discriminated most significantly of all between nonrelapsers and relapsers ($p < .001$), but only within informants' reports. (Unlike *SSA*, *SFA* measures satisfaction directly in its multiple-choice response format; see Appendixes E and F.) The corresponding free-time behavior measures, *FTA-P* (Free-Time Activities–Patient) and *FTA-I*, did not predict relapse significantly. But the clinical and social importance of onlookers' *satisfaction* with patients' free-time activities now stands out in bold relief throughout nearly all of the major analyses. Expectations may also be involved here as in *SSA*, though we have no psychometric documentation for this. What we do have is the highlighting of another area which calls for special attention on the part of aftercare counselors. With our patients' high unemployment rate, coupled with residuals and fluctuations of illness, it is understandable how their time at home may have hung heavily on others' hands if not on their own.

The *Psy* scale is a rather heterogeneous set of 24 items which do not load highly on any of the other 12 clusters embodied in the KAS informant Form R1 (Table I-2; Appendix F). Since it has shown superior sensitivity across the board, let us note what kind of patient it was describing. The following seven items were those most frequently endorsed by informants as having been observed "sometimes," "often," or "almost always" during Month 1:

I- 5. acts as if he has no interest in things;
I-12. feels that people don't care about him;
I-55. gets annoyed easily;
I-67. stays away from people;
I-71. prefers to be alone;
II- 4. very quick to react to something you say or do;
II-16. acts as if he can't get certain thoughts out of his mind.

The patient scoring high in *Psy* was thus likely to have been withdrawn, self-depreciating, irritable, and preoccupied. It is noteworthy that these are distinctly social liabilities which weigh heavily in the one most generally effective psychopathological variable.

The four adjustment variables which have yielded least in the way of significant results are *FTA-P*, *Exp* (Verbal Expansiveness), *Str-P*, and *Str-I*. *FTA-P* has been negative in all major analyses, and *FTA-I* has done little better; it is not clear whether these matching scales failed to register some essential aspects of free-time activity or whether perhaps there was simply a persisting behavioral stereotype among our patients in this area, little related to other aspects of adjustment process and outcome. The poor performance of *Exp* may relate to its badly skewed distribution at Month 1 (Table II-3); most of the other variables so skewed also did poorly in the analyses. *Str-P* and *Str-I* were new scales never before used; their low yield could derive from their preliminary status and might improve if the scales were refined along lines we have considered (Michaux, Gansereit, McCabe, and Kurland, 1967). Apart from this question, however, we suspect that stress effects are more likely to be registered, even via instruments such as the present ones, in designs where the time perspective is shorter than it typically was in this study. Figure V-1 below, with its accompanying text, is a case in point.

## PREDICTION FROM EARLY LIFE-SITUATION VARIABLES[3]

### *Main Results*

Once again there was a meager yield of useful predictive results from this set of 40 variables. Breadwinner contribution was the only one significantly predicting rehospitalization, at the .05 level. As Table V-4 shows, those patients who functioned as "sole or major" breadwinners at Month 1 were highly unlikely to become rehospitalized at any time during the year, but lesser contribution was not decisively prognostic. We have already established that prime breadwinners were less sick than other patients at Month 1 (Table III-9; in addition, this economically important social role may well have deterred families from initiating rehospitalization even if some breadwinners had seemed to need it.

Table V-4 lists also the five other variables which had the most nearly significant predictive discriminations; all *p* values were at the .20 level. Within this limitation, work and homemaking was by far the most fruitful area—as it has been in all major analyses except for prediction of outcome (Table IV-6). Generally, the more industrious and responsible patients were those somewhat less likely to become relapsers.

[3]Under this heading, two life-situation variables were untestable because of skewed distributions: (1) Busiest single work week—patient's report, and (2) same item—informant's report.

*Table V-4. Early Life Situation Variables Most Effectively Predicting Rehospitalization*

| Item | Nonrelapsers | | Relapsers | |
|---|---|---|---|---|
| | *N* | Per Cent | *N* | Per Cent |
| Work and homemaking | | | | |
| Employment: duration (Pt.,[a] $p < .20$): | | | | |
| No part of month | 66 | 76 | 41 | 85 |
| Part of month | 14 | 16 | 2 | 4 |
| All month | 7 | 8 | 5 | 10 |
| Employment: duration (Inf., $p < .20$): | | | | |
| No part of month | 66 | 76 | 41 | 85 |
| Part of month | 16 | 18 | 3 | 6 |
| All month | 5 | 6 | 4 | 8 |
| Breadwinner contribution (Inf., $p < .05$):[b] | | | | |
| No contribution | 52 | 67 | 31 | 67 |
| Less than major | 14 | 18 | 14 | 30 |
| Sole or major | 12 | 15 | 1 | 2 |
| Homemaker responsibility (Pt., $p < .20$):[b] | | | | |
| None, self only, or shared | 21 | 36 | 19 | 56 |
| Sole responsibility | 37 | 64 | 15 | 44 |
| Treatment | | | | |
| Where received (Pt., $p < .20$): | | | | |
| Nowhere (not in treatment) | 17 | 20 | 9 | 19 |
| Spring Grove OPC or other public clinic | 52 | 60 | 35 | 73 |
| All other: private doctor, etc. | 18 | 21 | 4 | 8 |
| Stress | | | | |
| "Good" event(s) during month (Pt., $p < .20$): | | | | |
| None | 35 | 40 | 27 | 56 |
| One or more | 52 | 60 | 21 | 44 |

[a]Respondent: Pt. (patient), Inf. (informant).

[b]Some cases excluded; see Appendix R.

## *Relation of Treatment to Rehospitalization*

The nine treatment variables are quite scantily represented in Table V-4. The single tabulated variable, "where received," shows very little difference in relapse-proneness between patients who at Month 1 were untreated and those who were attending public clinics; what difference does prevail is largely that which militates against relapse for patients in the "all other" category, most of whom were seeing private psychiatric or nonpsychiatric physicians. Moreover, if the comparison is limited only to treated patients, we find that the risk of relapse was over twice as great for those in public clinics (mostly the Spring Grove Outpatient Clinic) as for all others (seen mostly by private doctors); the difference is of borderline significance, $p < .10$. In the absence of random assignment to treatment, inference as to comparative therapeutic effectiveness is patently unwarranted. The observed trend is most likely associated with differential patient characteristcs, here undetermined, which were related to choice of Month-1 treatment facility.

As exhibited heretofore, for example in Table II-8, there were six life-situation items dealing with prescription and use of psychotropic medication–three questions answered by patients and informants independently. On the basis of Month-1 reports, none of them came near to predicting rehospitalization: probability levels approached chance expectations. Here again it is essential to keep in mind that, in our study, patients were not randomly assigned to the various groups.

Considering the Month-1 treatment evidence as a whole and in the context of other findings, we believe the results, as regards later rehospitalization experience, are most plausibly interpretable as follows: Drug-treated patients began the year somewhat sicker, at least by one criterion, than those without drugs (Table III-5). Presumably drugs operated to reduce their relapse potential, but only to a point where it approximately equaled that of patients who started the year without drugs. As for where treatment was received at Month 1 (Table V-4), the same interpretation is probably applicable to the similarity in relapse rates of the "nowhere" and "public clinic" groups.[4] The remaining patients, treated principally by private doctors, may have been subject to two conditions favoring their lower relapse rate: (1) less likelihood of being professionally advised to re-enter the hospital–in accord with our "surveillance" hypothesis as regards Spring Grove Clinic patients and (2) better in-community staying power in terms of personal resources, as reflected in their seeking the most expensive

[4]For present purposes, such rates are better indicated by percentages totaling horizontally instead of vertically as tabulated. So calculated, the relapse rates were: treated nowhere, 35 per cent; public clinics, 40 per cent; all other, 18 per cent.

private treatment in most instances. The surveillance effect may also have helped to account for the fact that public clinic patients did not have a lower relapse rate than those treated nowhere; in the Spring Grove Clinic, hospitalization and outpatient therapy tend to be subsumed together under a general concept of modulated patient care.

*Can Relapse-Prone Individuals Be Prognostically Identified?*

Having tested all of the project's standard variables as predictors of relapse within the year, we may now extract from our tables those most likely to prove useful to the aftercare clinician (subject to their replication). Eight such "prognostic signs" are available, discriminating at probability levels ranging from .05 to .001. Only the first two are based on pre-lease information; the remaining six pertain to patient behavior during the first 30 posthospital days and call for one factual inquiry plus administration of selected KAS measures to the patient and an informant. The eight most promising predictors are as follows:

| | Prognosis for nonrehospitalization within year | |
|---|---|---|
| Item | Favorable | Unfavorable |
| Diagnosis | other than schizophrenic | schizophrenic |
| No. of *prior* hospitalizations | 0 to 2 | 3 or more |
| Breadwinner contribution[5] | sole or major | less than major |
| KAS–Patient: | | |
| *SEA* | score 35 or more | score 34 or less |
| *SSA* | score 8 or less | score 9 or more |
| KAS–Informant: | | |
| *Psy* | score 36 or less | score 37 or more |
| *SSA* | score 6 or less | score 7 or more |
| *SFA* | score 30 or less | score 31 or more |

Given this information on an aftercare patient, the clinician could single out for special therapeutic attention the most ominously deviant signs among the last six listed. Further, by

[5]Limited to patients with dependents to be supported.

examining specific item responses in those KAS measures so chosen, he could proceed to pinpoint topics and activities suitable for focused concern in his counseling with the patient and/or informant.

## LONGITUDINALLY DISCERNIBLE PORTENTS OF REHOSPITALIZATION

Thus far we have dealt only with "cross-sectional" predictors of relapse, i.e., data collected at a single point in time prior to readmission. Within our project design it was also possible, via the concept of course of adjustment, to investigate potentially critical processes observable only in longitudinal perspective.

### *Adjustment Changes Portending Rehospitalization*

Suppose that a newly discharged patient is scheduled for monthly aftercare appointments and that he succeeds in remaining out of the hospital for six months. What can we learn about such patients' clinical course during that time that would warn us of the risk of later rehospitalization, or contraindicate such risk?

In our "complete" group there were 16 "late relapsers" who fitted the above description: Their first or only readmission did not occur until Month 7 or later. An appropriate comparison group were the 51 complete nonrelapsers whom we have already studied in Chapter III. If these two groups should show differential courses on any of the 26 adjustment variables during Months 1 through 6, results would be tentatively interpretable as prognostically meaningful vis-à-vis risk of later rehospitalization (Months 7 through 12).

Statistical procedure for determining differential courses was the same trend analysis as that used with the complete nonrelapsers, here applied separately to the two groups and with additional computations to test "*mean differences between groups* with respect to each trend component investigated. . . . The finding of a statistically significant *F*-ratio can be interpreted as meaning . . . different trends over time with respect to the variable analyzed in the population sample. Plotting the column means for each . . . group separately and comparing the resulting curves visually should reveal to the investigator the basis for any statistically significant finding" (Shaffer, Forbes, and DeFelice, 1967).

*F* tests of the 26 adjustment variables yielded very scanty significant results, not beyond overall chance expectations, for six-month linear trend differences between nonrelapsers and late relapsers. Only one variable, *Anx* (Anxiety), unequivocally discriminated in favor of nonrelapsers ($p < .05$). Nonrelapsers improved from a mean of 7.7 at Month 1 to 6.7 at Month 6, while late relapsers worsened from 7.1 at Month 1 to 7.5 at Month 6.

One additional variable, *SFA-P*, likewise discriminated by *F* test at the .05 level but the comparative longitudinal courses were anomalous: Late relapsers' satisfaction with their free-time activities improved *more* than did nonrelapsers'. Initial and final (Month-6) means for the former were 33.1 and 28.3; *t* for the linear trend was 2.51, $p < .05$. For the latter, initial and final means were 29.9 and 29.2 and the linear trend was nonsignificant. In other words, both groups apparently improved on this variable and the late relapsers' greater improvement was associated with a (nonsignificantly) worse initial status than nonrelapsers'. While this finding is provocative in its very oddness, we forego interpretive speculation, noting only that its pattern is unlike that of any of the other 23 KAS variables in this analysis.

Other aspects of the results, apart from the *F* tests for linear trend differences, proved at least highly suggestive as regards adjustment changes portending relapse. In particular there were six adjustment variables on which (1) nonrelapsers showed significant linear-trend improvement through Month 6, *but* (2) late relapsers deviated negligibly from a level "no change" course. The variables in question are those for which *p* values are shown in Table V-5: *LOE-P*, *Bel* (Belligerence), *Anx*, *Psy*, *Ner* (Nervousness), and *Hyp* (Hyperactivity). Worsening or nonimproving trends on these measures during the first six posthospital months, then, were closely associated with relapse during the remainder of the year. As sources for this kind of prognostic information, informants were somewhat more fruitful than patients. In terms of manifest

*Table V-5. Contrasting Longitudinal Tendencies, Nonrelapsers vs. Late Relapsers, Months 1 through 6*

| Variable | Contrasting Tendency | | | | Mean at Mos. 1, 6 | |
|---|---|---|---|---|---|---|
| | Linear *t* Test: *p* | | Average Change[a] | | | |
| | Nonrelapsers | Relapsers | Nonrelapsers | Relapsers | Nonrelapsers | Relapsers |
| KAS–Patient (see also Informant below): | | | | | | |
| *LOE-P*[b] | .05 | N.S. (.70) | | | 37.3, 39.0 | 36.8, 36.8 |
| *FTA-P* | | | –0.01 | 0.80 | 47.6, 47.4 | 48.6, 49.5 |
| KAS–Informant only: | | | | | | |
| *Bel* | .05 | N.S. (.30) | | | 4.5, 4.3 | 4.5, 4.2 |
| *Neg* | | | –0.56 | 0.29 | 12.1, 11.3 | 12.1, 12.1 |
| *Hel* | | | –0.45 | 0.01 | 5.7, 5.1 | 5.6, 5.8 |
| *Anx* | .01 | N.S. (.30) | –0.85 | 0.20 | 7.7, 6.7 | 7.1, 7.5 |
| *Psy* | .02 | N.S. (.30) | | | 33.8, 31.3 | 35.3, 34.3 |
| *Ner* | .05 | N.S. (.40) | | | 7.6, 6.8 | 7.6, 6.7 |
| *Biz* | | | –0.14 | 0.21 | 5.7, 5.5 | 5.9, 5.9 |
| *Hyp* | .01 | N.S. (.30) | | | 4.7, 3.9 | 4.9, 4.4 |
| *Sta*[b] | | | 0.19 | –1.86 | 30.0, 30.8 | 30.6, 28.5 |
| KAS–Informant (see also Patient above): | | | | | | |
| *SEA-I*[b] | | | 0.72 | –0.40 | 35.5, 36.7 | 34.8, 34.7 |
| *FTA-I* | | | –1.18 | 0.22 | 49.1, 47.5 | 50.6, 50.9 |

[a]Difference between Month-1 mean and composite mean of all scores on same scale for Months 2 through 6, in raw-score units.

[b]On these three adjustment variables only, high scores are favorable. Results must be interpreted accordingly.

content, psychopathological scales figured most densely, judgmental scales about as densely as in the total set of 26, and social scales not at all; it is primarily illness in the clinical sense that is involved in these longitudinal discriminations.

Another way to discover potentially meaningful tendencies in results from this computer program is to compare average change values for the two groups. Variables on which nonrelapsers improved and late relapsers worsened in this respect can be considered due for special attention in future studies of relapse, though less rigorously proved out than those heretofore noted. There were eight such measures: See Table V-5, "Average Change" columns.

In the right-hand section of the table are listed, mainly as supplemental information, initial and terminal means for all tabulated variables. It should be remembered that the results we have surveyed involved scores not only at these two months but also at the four intervening months.

*Anx* emerged in Chapter III as a variable repeatedly sensitive in analyses of course of adjustment; it was much less so thereafter in predictions of adjustment and rehospitalization from Month-1 scores. But here, where our focus was again (partly) on course of adjustment, *Anx* was again pre-eminently informative. It was the only variable discriminating between nonrelapsers and late relapsers by all three procedures: the $F$ test for differences in linear trends, the inspection of linear-trend $t$ tests, and the inspection of average changes.

On the other hand, the two stress indexes once again failed to register postulated differences. In fact, in the trend analyses they functioned quite contrarily: Trends for nonrelapsers were nonsignificant, while late relapsers' scores *improved* both on *Str-P* ($p < .05$) and *Str-I* ($p < .01$). Are we to infer that decreasing stress may predispose patients to rehospitalization? It would be a premature conclusion in view of the newness of our measuring instrument, but the question must certainly be left open. We suspect that its answer will depend on more detailed knowledge as to whether certain kinds or conditions of stress may be harmful while others may be helpful; the possibility that marital-sexual stress was helpful for our patients has already been noted in connection with

Table IV-6, and it could be that this kind of stress was more often reported by the subjects in this analysis.[6]

*Month-by-Month Adjustment Status as Related to Later Rehospitalization*

Built into the computer program here used was a procedure for separate analysis of each periodic set of repeated measurements of each variable: "In addition, possible differences between treatment groups can be investigated at each observational point by employing . . . a series of one-way analyses of variance across treatments at each observational point. . . . It will usually be found that the results of the . . . several analyses supplement one another so that logically satisfying conclusions can be drawn" (Shaffer, Forbes, and DeFelice, 1967).

*Table V-6. Significant Monthly Differences in Adjustment, Nonrelapsers vs. Late Relapsers, Months 1 through 6*

| Variable | Significant Results | | | | | | |
|---|---|---|---|---|---|---|---|
| | No. of Mos. Sig. | By Month No.: *p* | | | | | |
| | | 1 | 2 | 3 | 4 | 5 | 6 |
| KAS–Patient (see also Informant below): | | | | | | | |
| *SEA-P* | 2 | .025 | * | * | * | .025 | * |
| *SSA-P* | 1 | .05 | * | * | * | * | * |
| KAS–Informant only: | | | | | | | |
| *Neg* | 1 | * | .05 | * | * | * | * |
| *Hyp* | 1 | * | .05 | * | * | * | * |
| KAS–Informant (see also Patient above): | | | | | | | |
| *SSA-I* | 1 | * | * | .05 | * | * | * |
| *FTA-I* | 1 | * | * | .05 | * | * | * |
| *SFA-I* | 4 | .01 | .005 | .025 | * | * | .025 |

*Difference not significant.

[6]Results of the 52 linear-trend *t* tests (26 variables, 2 groups) have been presented only selectively. The complete inventory is as follows. Both groups improved significantly during the first six months on *Sym* and *LOE-I*. Only nonrelapsers improved significantly on the six variables so noted in Table CT; late relapsers did not change appreciably on them. Only late relapsers improved significantly (as we have reported) on *SFA-P*, *Str-P*, and *Str-I*. Neither group changed significantly on any of the remaining 15 variables: *SEA-P*, *SSA-P*, *FTA-P*, *Exp*, *Neg* (Negativism), *Hel* (Helplessness), *Sus*, *Wdl*, *Con*, *Biz*, *Sta*, *SEA-I*, *SSA-I*, *FTA-I*, and *SFA-I*.

In the present problem, this approach entailed 156 $F$ tests, comparing nonrelapsers with late relapsers on each variable at each of six months. Eleven of these were significant at or beyond the .05 level and are shown in Table V-6. The results do indeed supplement, and also extend, previous indications: Late relapsers' mean scores were worse than nonrelapsers' in each instance, and the discriminating variables were not limited to those already highlighted above. Notably, most of the significant differences occurred early in the year; only 2 of the 11 were later than Month 3. It is possible that adjustment *status* during the first few post-hospital months is at least as important for avoiding later relapse as is the early *course* of adjustment.[7] Four of the seven tabulated variables were among those previously found to predict, on the basis of Month-1 scores, relapse at any time after that month: *SEA-P*, *SSA-P*, *SSA-I*, and *SFA-I* (Table V-3).

## *Environmental Stress at Critical Points before Rehospitalization*

Scores on *Str-P* and *Str-I* were specially investigated in two supplemental analyses aimed at elucidating further the functions of these variables as precursors of rehospitalization. The first analysis was conducted while data collection was still in progress

[7]It may even be more important. In an extensive double series of analyses, covering as many relapsers as possible up to a maximum $N$ of 38, we tested each adjustment variable to answer two questions: (1) Taking Month 1 as the base measure and proceeding forward in time, at what pre-relapse month(s) did the mean differ significantly from the Month-1 mean? (2) Taking the "eleventh-hour" relapse test as the base measure and working *backward* in time, at what month(s) did the mean differ significantly from the relapse test mean? (The dual approach was in one sense necessitated by the temporally progressive attrition entailed in both directions via individual differences in length of pre-relapse in-community time.) The statistic used was the $t$ test for differences between correlated means. The yield from both series of analyses was clearly trivial by three standards considered jointly: (1) total number of significant month-to-month changes (nine), (2) direction of changes when significant (four in expected direction, five contrary to expected), and (3) magnitude of differences in mean scores (very small).

None of the significant changes occurred between the special Relapse Test and the last regular test preceding it; that is, there was no evidence of "eleventh-hour" worsening in adjustment such as might have been viewed as a precipitating factor in readmission. We should qualify this finding by restating two special features peculiar to the relapse test: (1) It was administered to both respondents shortly *after* the patient's readmission and was therefore, unlike the regular pre-relapse monthly tests, potentially subject to retrospective contamination. (2) Its time span was not the standard 30-day period; it covered whatever number of days had elapsed between the last prior regular test and the date of rehospitalization, and this number naturally varied from patient to patient.

and was therefore limited to groups smaller than usual. Complete results have been published separately (Michaux, Gansereit, McCabe, and Kurland, 1967) and are here only partly recapitulated.

Patient and informant stress-index scores were summed for each case and the total was used as the single variable to be studied. Equally sized groups of nonrelapsers and relapsers were matched identically on test-months to be analyzed, and as closely as possible on age, sex, marital status, and diagnosis. The one-tailed *t* test was used to compare group means so as to test the predictive hypothesis that stress would be inordinately high for relapsers at two points in time before they became rehospitalized: Month 1 and the latest regular test before readmission. Tests for both of these periods were cross-validated on samples designated "B." Results as graphed in Figure V-1 were as follows:

| Period | Sample | Mean Stress | | *p* |
|---|---|---|---|---|
| | | Nonrelapsers | Relapsers | |
| Month 1 | $A_1$ | 8.3 | 30.0 | .05 |
| Month 1 | $B_1$ | 25.7 | 34.3 | N.S. |
| Pre-relapse | $A_2$ | 15.0 | 35.0 | .025 |
| Pre-relapse | $B_2$ | 10.9 | 22.7 | Borderline (.10) |

Against the uneven and generally negative stress-index results heretofore reported, these partially corroborative findings must be accorded some weight in view of the more rigorous compilation of cases and scores. On the other hand, the undersized groups preclude considering results as definitive for the project as a whole.

*Pre-relapse Fluctuations in Environmental Stress*

Raw data for the second special study of stress were also hand-compiled to fit a predetermined schema. Again the two respondents' reports were pooled to obtain a single stress score; this time, cases were drawn from the entire sample of participants, but only relapsers were studied. As in other relapse analyses, only the first rehospitalization was considered in compiling scores.

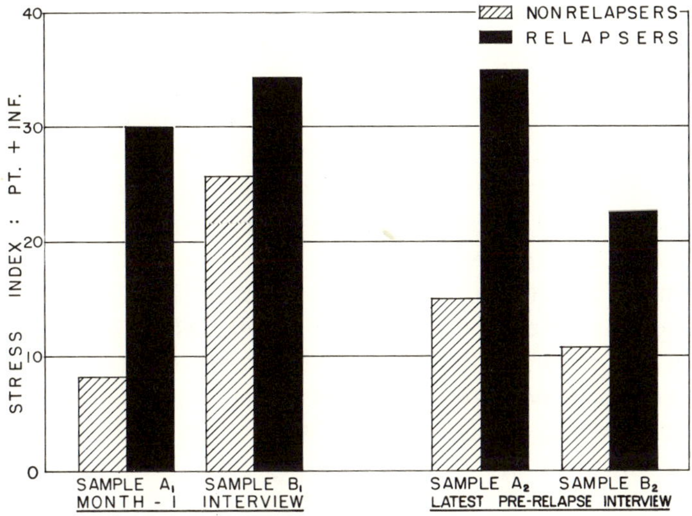


Figure V-1. Stress-index mean scores as predictors of rehospitalization. Results are for earliest (left) and latest (right) scores usable as predictors. Patient and informant scores were summed for each case and the totals were used as composite scores. Number of cases: Sample $A_1$–6 nonrelapsers, 6 relapsers; $B_1$–7, 7; $A_2$–10, 10; $B_2$–11, 11.

The question we posed was whether or not there had been clinically meaningful patterns of change or fluctuation in stress from Month 1 up to the time of rehospitalization. There were 26 relapsers whose data met three requirements for longitudinal adequacy: (1) The patient had remained out of the hospital for at least the first three months.[8] (2) Both respondents had completed the relapse test and also the last regular test before relapse. (3) Not more than one of the earlier pre-relapse tests had been missed by either or both respondents. (Test 1 was of course complete for everyone.)

It was found that, in order to educe meaningful patterns in any appreciable quantity, it was necessary to include the "eleventh-hour" relapse test in each case's series. Three patterns–A, B, and C–were postulated before inspecting the data. A fourth, D, was

[8]Four of the relapsers had remained in the community only through the first three months, the minimum required time. At the other extreme, seven had had from 8 to 11 months of unbroken in-community time.

later found unexpectedly. The patterns and their observed frequencies were as follows:

*A. No meaningful score sequence:* 12 cases, 46 per cent of total. We postulated this category on the ground that environmental stress could not be assumed to be a prepotent force in all relapses. It was defined in advance as "not classifiable B or C"; the definition was subsequently modified to exclude pattern D as well.

*B. Precipitating stress:* 9 cases, 34 per cent. This was the most frequent of the three meaningful patterns. The requirement was that the relapse test stress score should be higher than every earlier score in the series.

*C. Late and persisting stress increase:* 1 case, 4 per cent. The requirement was that the relapse test score must be equaled by one or more adjacently preceding scores and higher than the Month-1 score as well as any other earlier scores if present in a given series. Despite the single-case frequency, we feel that this pattern should be hypothetically retained in further studies.

*D. High initial and terminal stress:* 4 cases, 15 per cent. In consigning cases to A, B, or C we observed that four subjects had higher stress at Month 1 *and* on the relapse test than at any other pre-relapse months. This pattern, established by hindsight, was our earliest recognition of possible vulnerabilities peculiar to Month 1; only later did other indications of the first month's sensitivity become revealed as we assimilated our entire output of results.

On balance, then, about two-fifths of these 26 relapsers exhibited pre-relapse stress fluctuation patterns specified in advance as meaningful (B and C); if we include in the count the unexpected D pattern, the aggregate of cases with apparently meaningful patterns was slightly over one-half. These results constitute further tentative evidence that the stress index may elicit useful information by way of designs fashioned with close attention to its implications. The results do not, however, contraindicate the need for refinement of the interview technique. In the two auxiliary studies just presented, the combining of patient and informant stress scores may have functioned to some extent as a makeshift refinement, although complete results from the first study did not decisively support this notion.

## PHENOMENOLOGY OF REHOSPITALIZATION

Reappraising all of this chapter's information in the extended perspective of the study as a whole, we may now inferentially describe the process of our patients' rehospitalization in terms of what appear to be its essential clinical, psychosocial, and transactional features. The movement leading to rehospitalization is compounded of four interlocking conditions, each of which appears crucial in its own right. (1) A person who is not psychiatrically healthy undertakes to live among persons who, for the most part, are. (2) In so doing, he is additionally handicapped by the inordinate stresses of a sudden and drastic change in his own environment and social role, thereby becoming subject to exacerbation of his illness. (3) His sick behavior in turn perturbs those with whom he must live and interact—not only by way of their adverse episodic reactions, but also via their progressive disappointment as he fails to meet their expectations. (4) Those persons most closely affiliated with the patient, and hence most vulnerable to his interpersonal transgressions, are also, in our prevailing social structure, among those most eligible to become instrumental in his rehospitalization.

The time required for readmission to become a finality must vary with innumerable circumstances of patient-environment interaction. To the extent that endogenous psychobiological processes are involved in any patient's illness, they constitute a fifth contributory condition. It is a condition not always respected by socially oriented investigators; an exception is the study of rehospitalized schizophrenics by Reilly, Wilson, and McClinton (1967), who speculated that "at least in some of these patients, hospitalization may be dealing with symptomatic peaks of disease of variable intensity that is little affected by outside influences."

Any treatment program which aims to prevent hospitalization must, we believe, take into account all four of the conditions we have formulated, plus the possible fifth. It must seek to help not only the patient but also his close affiliates. Table V-3 provides some of the specifics for those doing the work. In helping the patient, the program must not stop with treating his symptoms, no matter how potent the drug or other agent; it must enable him to flourish by active, self-originated, socially constructive modes of living. It must also deal with the gap between his own picture of his social performance and his self-expectations, especially when that gap is large.

As for the patient's "significant others," the effort to prevent hospitalization must assume that they are no less individually important than the patient himself in the healing and enabling process. In the foreground of their therapeutic involvement, the question of their unfolding perceptions of the patient must be kept open and personally meaningful to them. As persons with the difficult mission of living with a convalescing relative or close friend, they too will need special help in handling their expectations of the patient and their disappointments with him. Here again, the emphasis needs to be not merely on asymptomatic patient behavior; what appears cardinally important to the affiliate is the patient's *positive* mental health, his social reward value to himself and to others, his use of his free time as a commodity for self-enhancement and not as a decaying surplus which, unless absorbed, can clutter their lives.

## SUMMARY

The five background variables which best predicted rehospitalization during the posthospital year were education, number of prior hospitalizations, years hospitalized before last admission, diagnosis, and type of release. Schizophrenics were more often readmitted than nonschizophrenics, and convalescent-leave patients more than those discharged outright. Relapsers were comparatively low in education and had more and longer prior hospitalizations than nonrelapsers.

On the 26 measures of adjustment at Month 1, relapsers' averages were generally worse than nonrelapsers'. However, only the social and, especially, judgmental variables were dense among the significant predictors of rehospitalization. The four adjustment variables which have now proved most informative throughout all major analyses are *SEA-P*, *Psy*, *SSA-I*, and *SFA-I*.

On the whole the 40 life-situation variables functioned ineffectively as relapse predictors from Month-1 status. Breadwinners usually remained in the community all year, and other variables in the work and homemaking area discriminated with low effectiveness in the direction of less likelihood of relapse for patients who were comparatively industrious and responsible.

There were 16 "late relapsers" who remained unrehospitalized for the first six months and completed enough tests during that time to permit longitudinal comparisons with the 51 "complete nonrelapsers." *Anx* was the single most sensitive adjustment variable registering contrasting courses in the two groups during Months 1 through 6; nonrelapsers improved quite significantly by trend-analysis *t* test, while relapsers had a nonsignificantly worsening trend. On five other variables both groups improved but only the nonrelapsers' improvement was significant: *LOE-P*, *Bel*, *Psy*, *Ner*, and *Hyp*. When group differences were tested at each month independently, nonrelapsers averaged significantly better on 7 variables in 11 separate tests.

The two matching measures of environmental stress, *Str-P* and *Str-I*, have performed unevenly and generally uninformatively throughout all major analyses—in part, no doubt, because of their newness and their need for psychometric refinement. They appeared more promising in this chapter in two ancillary investigations which had been designed specifically to explore problems of stress in relation to rehospitalization.

Viewed in the perspective of all of the study's results, rehospitalization is understandable as the culmination of deteriorating interactions between the returning patient and his social environment. The patient is a troubled and stressed person at the outset, and his close affiliates become progressively perturbed by his sick behavior and by their own disappointment with him. Our findings unquestionably indicate that, for patients similar to ours, any effort to prevent hospitalization needs to deal therapeutically not only with the sick individual but also with those who share his daily living; and not only with arresting the patient's symptoms, but also, perhaps even more importantly, with enabling him to achieve enduring social and recreational rewards. And, apart from the patient's actual behavior, effective help must hold recurrently in focus what he expects of himself, what others expect of him, and the discrepancy between expectations and performance.

Chapter VI

# Retrospect and Prospect

To close the report, we shall relax our grip on the specifics of results and immediate interpretations and, at a higher, synoptic level, consider the study's net-balance yield. As in any such stock-taking, we must look both backward and forward—at the completed work, and at the unfolding future of mental health professions and programs.

Apart from its substantive findings, the project should be reconsidered also in terms of its trial demonstration of new methods. Concluding remarks on method and related topics are presented in Appendix U. The fact that our methodological ventures were in our judgment reasonably successful has, of course, considerable bearing on what we believe to be the usefulness of the project's results.

## TREATMENT PROGRAMS AND POLICIES

For public-health agents and planners, a number of issues have emerged from the study that will need to be reconsidered at choice-points in the designing of new clinical facilities and the planning of community and regional programs. Where does the hospital fit functionally in a comprehensive array of services? For whom is inpatient treatment essential and to whom should it be denied? Upon leaving the mental hospital, what kinds of patients will need what kinds of services? We would suggest that *local* studies somewhat like our own could contribute definitively to such decisions—in almost the same sense that local norms are often best for decisions based on psychological test scores. Such local studies, however, should certainly be more than replications of the present one. They might advantageously include patients admitted to, and/or discharged from, more than one facility; outpatient as well as inpatient treatment could be represented in the patient samples; and data could be collected continuously and cumulatively with no fixed end-point, for periodic analysis and evaluation. Studies so designed would constitute, in effect, operations research aimed at optimizing the effectiveness of an entire treatment system. The feasibility of repeatedly evaluating patients in their natural in-community habitats has been satisfactorily demonstrated by our project. We have shown that frequent, long-term clinical testing and interviewing for research purposes can be accomplished in conjunction with outpatient treatment visits, or in respondents' homes, or in a hospital—by workers not previously known to the subjects. The sensitive, personal nature of the information solicited poses no general difficulty. Electronic equipment and procedures for storing and processing such data on a large-scale public health basis are even now at an advanced stage of development in Maryland (Gorwitz, Bahn, Chandler, and Martin, 1963). Probably the major obstacle to their use in such research is the very real issue of confidentiality which, while comfortably handled in our study, assumes larger proportions with the storing of personalized evaluative data in a public service register.

At lower service echelons, those most likely to find new points of departure in this investigation are on-line clinicians and researchers working in aftercare, in community mental health, and in programs offering alternatives to hospitalization. In our sample, four patients out of five began the posthospital year with some form of outpatient care. Clearly, a conscientious effort was made by Spring Grove and its outpatient service to provide continuing treatment as needed—at least for the newly released patient, though as the year progressed the treatment picture became questionable in regard to discontinuance of chemotherapy for those patients who were thereafter rehospitalized. Does an aftercare program such as Spring Grove's represent a wise investment of the considerable professional time and skills involved? It would be hard to defend outright an affirmative answer in view of the high rehospitalization rates observed not only in our own sample but in many others. One must still grant the legitimacy of complaints such as the one voiced in a letter we recently received from the superintendent of a large out-of-state public mental hospital. He had just finished a cohort study of patient movement disclosing oft-repeated hospitalization for many (Peterson and Olson, 1964). With an outlook far from sanguine, he wrote to us: "It seems to us that either we [in hospitals] are not treating patients well enough to cure them or, if we are doing fairly well, a lot of planning is going on not taking into consideration that chronic patients do continue to develop. As people on the receiving end of this planning, we find some of it quite alarming."[1]

## THE HOSPITAL'S PREDICAMENT

The new breed of community-centered clinicians, with their repertoires of innovative treatments, offer one hope of relief and betterment. But the issue is not just prevention of hospitalization; what is at stake is the hypertrophied boundary between the mental hospital and the community it serves. For many years we could blame the hospital's isolation on the public's rejection of the mentally ill. But the advent of lay enlightenment and the burgeoning of the community mental health movement[2] can conceivably leave us so preoccupied with *preventing* hospitalization that the hospital's old dilemma may persist with only a different guise: we may end by failing to accord hospitals an integral function in the new system of comprehensive services. Mechanick and Nathan (1965) have already warned that: "Just as sole reliance on hos-

[1]Donald B. Peterson, personal communication, 1963. Quoted by permission.

[2]The optimism here must be qualified. The community mental health movement, like the mental hospital, is not immune from public ostracism. We know first-hand of one effort to open community services, not far from our own place of work, which encountered very serious neighborhood resistance. The same kind of opposition has been observed elsewhere (Kandel and Williams, 1964, pp. 39-40).

pitalization has provided one kind of rigid attitude, so then, the avoidance of hospitalization can also represent another kind of inflexibility."

As we try to deal with the uncertainty that besets the mental hospital's future, we must acknowledge that its isolation from the community it serves has been not only social (and frequently geographical) but also clinical: Only schematically, and rarely in actual practice, has the hospital been functionally continuous with other psychiatric services. Transactionally, hospitalization has represented more of a calamity to be dreaded than a constructive measure to be appropriately taken; an all-or-none, last-ditch reflex rather than a deliberate act. Nor has separatism been limited to admission practices. Too often, whenever a patient either enters or leaves the hospital, there occurs a sort of ceremonial washing of hands by those who are being relieved of responsibility for him. This division of labor is sustained and reinforced by traditional and legal guidelines for commitment, guardianship, and so on. It may seem helpful for those responsible; but what does it do for the patient? It means that he must live alternately in two worlds, all the while with an impaired sense of belonging in either. A person already sick must repeatedly readjust to two radically different environments, like a soldier returning to civilian life or an astronaut landing on the moon.

The point is by no means foreign to the heart of this study. Movement *into*, or *out of*, the hospital may entail serious environmental stress for the individual. But in the study, our admittedly limited effort to take direct account of all in-community stresses in our patients' life situations may well have failed to register adequately the stress of returning home, both at Month 1 and later when relapsers were again discharged throughout the study year.[3] It is therefore an open question as to how much contributory weight this particular kind of adversity may have carried in the inferior adjustment manifested by relapsers throughout the post-

[3]There were, however, some distinct intimations of the newly returned patient's sensitive position. At Month 1, a woman reported that a former friend had "snubbed" her. In another case an informant, when asked the question as to whether anything good had happened for the patient at Month 1, told the examiner: "Friends and relatives have accepted her readily and included her in activities" (Michaux, Gansereit, McCabe, and Kurland, 1967).

hospital year (Table III-6). Hence the notion that inpatient treatment per se may have harmed our patients must be qualified by the possibility that the special environmental pressures of returning home were, in their own right, decisively detrimental. Nevertheless, those particular pressures would not have existed without hospitalization. Devoting more clinical attention to such pressures, in pre- and post-discharge work with individual patients, would go hand in hand with relieving the functional isolation of inpatient treatment.[4]

## THE CLINICIAN'S ALTERNATIVES

Proponents of day hospitals and night hospitals often argue that their services have the advantage of not totally removing the patient from his accustomed living situation. It is true that the day or night hospital patient can live at home for half of each day. Does this condition spare him the experience of uprooting that comes at the start and finish of round-the-clock hospitalization? Perhaps so, but the converse is possible and needs to be investigated: At least for some patients, in some situations, partial hospitalization may be experienced as *daily* uprooting.

Implicit in much of what we have said is the need not merely for more appropriate and more effective services to patients but rather for greatly improved accuracy in clinical decision-making. Subjective, extemporized judgments about what to do next will clearly no longer suffice (if ever they have). There are now too many sprawlingly diverse facilities each representing a possible treatment choice—hospitals, home visitors, outpatient clinics, and so on; with each facility offering its own services—for example, drugs, social casework, behavior modification, and group psychotherapy; and, inside of each service, with still further differ-

[4]To support the notion of the stressfulness of emergence from isolation, there is provocative evidence from controlled laboratory experiments with dogs: See Fuller (1967).

The hospital's isolation needs also to be attacked by research—as has been attempted not only in the present study but also by Katz, Lowery, and Cole (1965) in their testing of relations between in-community and in-hospital measures of schizophrenics' behavior.

Some highly pertinent thoughts on the mission of research in community mental health have been advanced by Guy, Hogarty, and Gross (1965).

entiated choices to be made—such as how frequently and how intensively to treat.

Increased effectiveness in treating mental illness cannot be predicated simply on repertoire diversification. Now more than ever, the clinician needs to know, in standard and replicable terms, (1) the nature and severity of his patient's condition, and (2) for such a patient, what benefit, if any, is to be expected from available alternatives of therapeutic action. The manifold promises of community mental health cannot be truly fulfilled until research can provide the clinician with fairly explicit predictive guidelines, at least for his most frequent and most crucial treatment decisions.

If the proliferating community mental health services are not to become a muddle in which we lose our sense of therapeutic direction, we must therefore evaluate—and without delay—the comparative effectiveness of the various new treatment modalities and their differential suitability for various types of patients. The need for such research is not limited to the mental health field; it has been proclaimed more generally by a National Health Survey official: "Only on the basis of precise data with increasing scope and detail can advances in medical science and enlightened public policy be translated into decent health care for the entire population" (Linder, 1966). Some starts have been made for psychiatric patients, as in the Maryland work of Hogarty and associates who have used the KAS and other assessment techniques in a community mental health context (Hogarty, Katz, and Lowery, 1967; Hogarty, Guy, and Gross, 1968).

## PATIENTS AND AFTERCARE

Like Hogarty's work, the present study has sought to sharpen the sense of direction of those concerned with treatment refinements and innovations. It has provided (for example, in Figure II-1 and in Tables III-6, III-13, V-3, and V-6) a set of plausible interlocking findings which can serve as normative expectations for certain posthospital patients to whom certain aftercare treatments are available. Also, in normative terms, the study has enabled the aftercare clinician to gauge objectively the adjustment status of his patients (Appendix T). So equipped, as he monitors patients' ongoing conditions, he can act more discerningly in modulating treatment, planning environmental intervention, and so on. In such actions he may also take note of our disclosures pertaining to concurrent environmental stress and other aspects of patients' life situations (Table III-9, etc.).

More generally, as regards treatment policy, the study has yielded several pointed suggestions. Perhaps the two which best bear restatement are: (1) the advisability of counseling close relatives against holding inordinately high and tenacious expectations as to patients' posthospital performance, and (2) the distinct possibility that repeated hospitalization may do patients more harm than good. When relatives look to rehospitalization to relieve their growing disappointment with patients, the starting point for help should be to deal with their disappointment, and the patient-relative relationship which engendered it.

In still broader perspective, we would hope that the study has brought us somewhat closer to answering the kinds of urgent questions posed by other Maryland researchers: "Have our new treatment methods and concepts actually reduced the chronicity among patients, or have they merely substituted in-and-out movement for an extended hospitalization? What are the advantages and disadvantages in decreasing the length of [hospital] stay to a minimum when there is a high probability of subsequent readmission? Is the reduction achieved in total number of days of hospitalization of benefit to the patient and his family, or are patients being released prematurely?" (Gorwitz, Bahn, Klee, and Solomon, 1966). The questions echo the apprehensions of our correspondent, the state hospital superintendent quoted earlier. They cannot be answered by studies focused only on the hospital, or only on outpatient treatment; they demand of the researcher the comprehensive continuum-of-services approach. "We must all hang together, or assuredly we shall all hang separately"—as an eighteenth-century American scientist put it in the heat of political crisis.

Whether or not a patient needs aftercare upon leaving the hospital will clearly depend, in part, on how he has responded to inpatient treatment. In the best clinical practice, both questions—response to prior treatment and need for further help—are posed conjointly during pre-discharge planning. Realistically, the aftercare decision for each patient must, of course, be made in terms of whatever services are currently and locally available. At the same time, however, if it is felt that the aftercare service chosen for a particular patient holds less therapeutic promise than would some other specifiable mode of treatment *not* available then and there, it would be well to take note of the necessary compromise that is being made. Systematic serial compilation of such unmet needs within officially defined treatment sectors could provide data useful for planning new services in the sectors in question.

The problem of patients' readiness for hospital discharge is, as we are suggesting, far from simple. Hogarty has attacked it from the standpoint of individual patient assessment, devising a "Discharge Readiness Inventory" (Hogarty, 1966) and using it to investigate hospital release in relation both to patient readiness and to aftercare availability (Hogarty, 1968). As we consider the question's ramifications, the need is seen for a quite different but complementary assessment technique–a "Hospitalization Readiness Inventory," perhaps similar to the KAS, which would take stock of assets and liabilities in a patient's community adjustment and lend a quality of deliberation and thoroughness to a decision that is too often compelled by crisis, anxiety, and expediency. Our findings contain points of departure for developing such an inventory.

Let us look again at the Spring Grove patients we have studied. From the evidence on hand, they seem for the most part to have been not unready to leave the hospital. Their early posthospital adjustment averaged about as close to normal as one could reasonably hope for (Figure II-1). A substantial number of them avoided rehospitalization for a full year and tended to improve or at the very least not to worsen during that time (Table III-13). Yet others, also in substantial numbers, did become rehospitalized (Table III-1) and manifested a comparatively unfavorable posthospital course (Table III-6).

What can be surmised as to the appropriateness and effectiveness of the aftercare received by many patients in our cohort? Considering their apparently good early posthospital adjustment, one could argue that it was overdone (though such an argument would have to deal with the proposition that gains made by hospitalization may need to be maintained by outpatient treatment). But in terms of posthospital course and outcome one must admit that, at least for the less fortunate patients, there was *de facto* much room for improvement in aftercare effectiveness. Beyond this the design of the study is of course not such as to justify either acclaiming or impugning the particular varieties of aftercare which these particular patients received. The evidence does yield, however, some implicit suggestions for making aftercare more beneficial. More *clinical* attention needs to be paid to the patient's "significant other," typically the spouse or parent, who often figures as a prime decision-maker or decision-engenderer as regards the patient's treatment. This person's view of the patient's adjustment, as well as his degree of satisfaction therewith, clearly augurs and reflects much with reference to course and outcome (see especially Tables III-6 and V-3). Clinicians should be mindful that the relative's perceptions, as well as his judgments, of the patient are subject to therapeutic modification—and so are also his expectations, as previously noted.

The same evidence calls also for increased emphasis on *positive* mental health as a goal of treatment and as a force working counter to rehospitalization. We refer here to the kinds of socially desirable activities and judgments that are embodied in KAS measures *SEA* (Performance of Socially-Expected Activities), *LOE* (Level of Expectations), *SSA* (Satisfaction with Socially-Expected Activities), *FTA* (Free-Time Activities), and *SFA* (Satisfaction with Free-Time Activities). We do not mean to imply that symptoms of illness can safely be ignored, but rather that, in a treatment era when drugs are heavily relied on, clinical emphasis may have gravitated too much toward symptom reduction and too little toward the fostering of social well-being and effectiveness (Bonstedt and Akdogu, 1966). Where in-community improvement was most clearly discernible in our patients (Table III-13), it was registered more in terms of symptom reduction than of better social functioning. But, when rehospitalization was in focus, social behavior became more decisive (Tables III-6 and V-3), although symptoms of sickness did not cease to assert themselves (Table V-5).

Future research must inform the clinician more precisely about the social dynamics of rehospitalization. To function helpfully in averting or in recommending it, he especially needs further research-based insight into the role of the patient's family in that transaction (Clausen and Yarrow, 1955). High research priority should be given to elucidating the relations *between* symptomatic behavior and social performance, *between* endogenous (illness) factors and environmental conditions—both in the patient's community experience and in his avoidance of, or need for, rehospitalization. Study of those very important relations should particularly take into account two processes which we believe hold much to be learned because their involvement is so clearly both symptomatic and social, both endogenous and environmental: They are environmental stress (Table III-13: Figure V-1) and the patient's work and homemaking activity (Tables III-8, III-9, III-10, and V-4).

During the many months of work on this project, we devoted studious attention to the voluminous literature of relevant research and commentary by other investigators. Our citations have barely skimmed the surface of that rich body of readings. (The new modality of family therapy, obviously fraught with potentials in this area, has been bypassed in our report.) There is much to be gleaned by any reader who can delve deeply enough to cross-check our findings with others. By considering particularly the points of divergence and apparent contradiction, he will come upon additional issues for treatment and research which merit attention equally with those we have discussed.

## SUMMARY

Some of the study's broader implications are educed as they pertain to problems faced by public-health agents, mental-health program planners, clinicians, and research workers. Important issues are the transitional state of today's mental hospital, the manifold decisions the clinician must make in treatment, and the need to maximize the effectiveness of aftercare.

In regard to aftercare, the need is pointed up for closer clinical attention to the social and family dynamics of rehospitalization and its prevention. Both in treatment and in research, patient-relative interactions merit high priority for action. So likewise does the problem of deliberately and objectively assessing patients' readiness for hospitalization. Greater emphasis in aftercare may need to be placed on fostering the patient's positive mental health, as opposed to merely reducing his symptoms.

# Appendixes*

*An asterisk designates each appendix (or section within an appendix) dealing primarily with methodology, for the benefit of readers interested in this aspect of the study, but of less interest to readers who concentrate on its clinical and social aspects.

Appendix A

# *Letter Requesting Patient's and Informant's Participation

This letter was mailed to each eligible patient on or about the 25th day after the patient had left the hospital. It set the proposed time for the first monthly evaluation, on approximately the 30th posthospital day. To guard against violating the patient's privacy, the return address on the envelope was shown as "Box 3235, Survey Office, Baltimore 28, Maryland."

---

Form LS-9A

FRIENDS OF PSYCHIATRIC RESEARCH, INC.
SPRING GROVE STATE HOSPITAL
BALTIMORE 28, MARYLAND

[Date]

________________________

________________________

________________________

Dear ________ :

We are conducting a community follow-up survey of people who, like yourself, have recently been patients at Spring Grove. The main purpose of the survey is to learn how people get along after leaving the hospital, in order to improve the care and treatment of future patients. Persons who take part in the survey will be asked a set of questions about what they have been doing and how they have felt since leaving Spring Grove. All information will be confidential. It will be collected and used only by the Research Department, and not by the hospital treatment staff.

We are asking each person to visit our Survey Office for about one hour, and to bring with him (or her) an adult relative who has been in close touch with him during the past few weeks. We have scheduled an appointment for you and your relative as follows:

TIME: ________________

PLACE: Hamilton Building–please use the Outpatient Clinic entrance

REPORT TO: Receptionist, who will notify Mrs. Doretha Brown, Secretary.

It is necessary for a relative to come with you in order for the survey procedures to be completed. There will be no charge for this visit.

We realize that coming here may involve some inconvenience and expense for you and your relative. Because of this, we are willing to reimburse you to the total extent of $5.00 if you need this assistance. (This amount can be increased if your actual expenses in keeping the appointment are more than $5.00.)

We also realize that you and your relative may not be able to visit us at the particular time we have scheduled. If you would prefer a different appointment time, or if you have any questions, please call Mrs. Brown at 744-3182. We will accept "collect" long-distance calls.

By taking part in our survey, you and your relative will be doing a real service to mental health research in its effort to discover better ways to help patients and prevent psychiatric hospitalization. Please keep this letter and show it to the receptionist when you arrive at Hamilton Building.

Sincerely yours,

William W. Michaux, Ph.D.
Survey Co-ordinator

WWM/dmb

Appendix B

# *Project Information Given to New Participants

The following material, in leaflet form, was ordinarily given to the patient just after Test 1, when the Project Director or Examiner explained the 12-month project schedule and requested participation for the remaining 11 months. The informant, who was usually present with the patient, was told that he or she might also want to read the leaflet.

---

## THE COMMUNITY FOLLOW-UP SURVEY

This information is for ex-patients of Spring Grove State Hospital who are taking part in our survey.

We have answered here the questions that people most often ask us about the survey. However, after reading this you may still have other questions that we haven't covered here. If so, please let us know.

1. *WHAT IS THE PURPOSE OF THE SURVEY?*

The main purpose of the Community Follow-up Survey is to help doctors, nurses, and social workers learn more about how patients get along after they leave the hospital. This will help us to improve the treatment we give in the hospital, the outpatient clinics, and the day centers. In the long run, it will help to keep people out of the hospital.

2. *WHAT GOOD WILL THE SURVEY DO* ME?

If you happen to need treatment in the future, you will get the benefit of what we learn from the survey. Perhaps you will also get some satisfaction from knowing that, by answering our questions, you have done your share to help other patients. Furthermore, the questions that we ask you may give you some helpful ideas about handling your own problems, by showing you what your strong points are, and what points may need further improvement.

3. *WHAT WILL BE DONE WITH THE INFORMATION I GIVE ABOUT MYSELF?*

You are one of 100 people we are studying. All of them are former patients of Spring Grove. The information will be very carefully analyzed and studied by trained research scientists, who will write technical reports telling what has been learned from the survey. These reports will be published in professional mental health journals, where they can be read by any worker, anywhere, in the mental health field. Therefore, in the long run, the information you give us will be helpful not only for the staff at Spring Grove, but for many other people in the fields of psychiatry, psychology, and social work.

4. *WILL THE INFORMATION I GIVE BE CONFIDENTIAL?*

Yes. Your name will not be used; your records will be given a special number to be used instead of your name. If anyone asks to see our information on you, we must get your own written permission before releasing it. It will not be put in your Spring Grove treatment file, and will not be seen by anyone who is or was responsible for your treatment.

5. *CAN THE INFORMATION I GIVE BE USED AGAINST ME IN ANY WAY?*

Absolutely not.

6. *WILL THE APPOINTMENT TAKE A LONG TIME?*

No. The average time is about an hour. Some people finish in 30 minutes; others may take an hour and a half.

7. *WHO ELSE WILL BE THERE WHEN I COME FOR MY APPOINTMENT?*

You and your relative will be seen privately. No one else will have an appointment at the same time. Your Examiner will be a Research Assistant who has college training in psychology and mental hygiene. A doctor will be available in case either you or your Examiner should have any questions.

8. *DO I HAVE TO COME TO SPRING GROVE FOR MY APPOINTMENT?*

Not necessarily. We can visit you and your relative at home if you prefer. Or, if you have an Outpatient Clinic appointment, either at Spring Grove or at another clinic, we may be able to arrange to see you and your relative when you visit the clinic.

9. *WHAT IF I AM NOT ABLE TO KEEP MY APPOINTMENT?*

Call 744-3182 in Baltimore and ask for the Follow-up Survey Secretary. We will be glad to schedule a different time for you. If you have to phone long-distance to reach us, we will accept a "Collect" call.

10. *WHY DO I HAVE TO ASK A RELATIVE TO TAKE PART IN THE SURVEY?*

Your relatives, who see you every day and share in your experiences, are the people who know most about how you are getting along. Of course you yourself can tell us a great deal, but a relative will often notice things that you may overlook. Research has already proved that a relative's report is a very useful source of personal information, even when the patient's own report about himself is also available.

11. *WHAT IS THE "RESEARCH DEPARTMENT"?*

The Research Department is a large group of scientists and technicians at Spring Grove who are conducting investigations in psychiatry and mental hygiene. The Community Follow-up Survey is one of many such studies now in progress. Other studies are concerned with alcoholic patients at the hospital, with finding the best drugs to treat mental illness, and with developing better methods of diagnosing, understanding, and treating psychiatric patients. Since 1953, when the Research Department was organized, we have published more than 80 articles reporting our findings and experiences. Our work is financed partly by the State of Maryland and partly by grants from the National Institute of Mental Health and from drug manufacturers. Our administrative and financial business is managed by Friends of Psychiatric Research Inc., a private, nonprofit, tax-exempt agency founded in 1955 by a group of Baltimore citizens.

12. *WHAT IF I HAVE OTHER QUESTIONS THAT HAVEN'T BEEN ANSWERED HERE?*

Your Examiner will either answer your questions or tell you where you can get the answers. If you need an answer before you see your Examiner, call 744-3182 in Baltimore and ask for the Follow-up Survey Secretary.

Appendix C

# *Complete Research Action Notes on One Case

These dated narrative notes were entered by various project staff members in the patient's research case file. Most of them were written by the secretary or the examiners who worked with the patient and her informant. The notes were recorded in the "Action Taken" section of Form LS-7, Actions Taken and Scheduled; a blank copy of this form is exhibited in Appendix D. The only changes we have made in reproducing the original notes below have been to remove superfluous matter, conceal identities of persons not on the project staff, and clarify what was being reported.

We have chosen this particular specimen case because of the diversity and representativeness of its logistical problems. Not all of our cases posed as many complications in data collection as this one—although quite a few did. The notes illustrate the kind of painstaking observations, staff actions, *and records* that proved essential to fulfill systematic research requirements in the face of uncontrollable variations in the patient's and informant's life situations.

The following are among the major problems in logistics exemplified by this case (dates indicate points of occurrence):

(1) co-ordinating research appointments with the patient's outpatient clinic aftercare appointments (6-9-64, 6-10-64, 7-8-64; 8-19-64 through 8-21-64, 10-7-64);

(2) obtaining an informant when there was no relative of the patient who could be expected to serve in this capacity (6-9-64, 6-10-64, 3-19-65);

(3) continuing data collection despite loss of the original informant (7-14-64 through 8-10-64);

(4) the occasional scrapping of obtained data in order to keep the timing of monthly evaluations within reasonable limits (9-17-64);

(5) some of the operational challenges posed by the patient's relapse: note especially in this case the untenableness of a neutral observer role by the research staff (3-15-65 through 3-17-65a);

(6) our efforts–in this instance not successful–to make a suitable referral for emergency clinical help (3-15-65a through 3-17-65b);

(7) the administration of the special relapse test, required by the research design, to evaluate adjustment in the period between the last regular test and rehospitalization (3-17-65a; 3-18-65 through 3-24-65);

(8) the research staff's obligation to conform to clinical-administrative requirements, even when these were extraneous to research objectives (3-23-65, 3-24-65);

(9) the necessity of periodic checks on the rehospitalized patient to make sure of resuming monthly research evaluations if the patient should return home during her study year (4-7-65 through 5-7-65a).

In this case, the patient was a 38-year-old female who was separated from her husband. She was living in Baltimore; neither of her two children lived with her. She had had eight psychiatric hospitalizations covering a total of five years; had a diagnosis of schizophrenic reaction, paranoid type; and was on convalescent leave from Spring Grove when she entered our study.

---

6-5-64. Sent patient initial letter requesting participation.

6-9-64. Tried to contact patient by phone. Talked with Mrs. Joan Martin, with whom patient used to live. Mrs. Martin said patient was not living with her now. She is residing somewhere in Randallstown, but Mrs. Martin did not know with whom she was living or the address. She said that if patient had an Outpatient Clinic appointment (here at hospital) she would probably keep it. We will try to see patient after she has seen her OPC doctor.

6-9-64a. Patient phoned to ask about research appointment. M.K.H. will call her back.

6-9-64b. Called patient who did not receive letter but did agree to see us Wednesday, 6-10-64 at 3:30 p.m. (after OPC visit at 3:00 p.m.) for Test 1. No informant will be with her. We will try to arrange for informant after patient arrives.

6-10-64. Patient reported for Test 1 after OPC visit. Unexpectedly, she was accompanied by a friend, Mrs. Rogers, who was able to serve as informant. Both agreed to see us again, Thursday, 7-16-64 at 3:30 p.m. here, after next clinic visit. Mrs. Barry (patient) will move in with Mrs. Rogers very soon. See Special Notes for address.

7-8-64. Patient called to change appointment from 7-16-64 to Tuesday, 7-14-64 at 3:30 p.m. here after OPC visit.

7-13-64. Called patient to confirm scheduled appointment for Test 2 here at 3:30 p.m. Tuesday, 7-14-64, after her OPC appointment. Mrs. Rogers will serve as informant.

7-14-64. Patient and informant completed Test 2 as scheduled after OPC visit. Both agreed to Test 3, Friday, 8-7-64 at 3:00 p.m. after 2:30 p.m. OPC visit. Mrs. Rogers will serve as informant even though patient now plans to move to a residence other than hers. (Check new address and phone at next session.)

8-7-64. Patient reported for Test 3 by herself after OPC visit. Former informant could not be reached. Patient agreed to Test 4 Friday, 9-11-64, at 2:45 p.m. after 2:30 p.m. OPC visit. Will try to arrange for new informant.

8-10-64. Called Mrs. King, with whom patient is now living. She agreed to serve as informant. Scheduled an appointment for Friday, 8-14-64, at 11:00 a.m. at her home. Informant only.

8-14-64. Completed Test 3, informant only, at Mrs. King's home. Very cooperative and interested informant. She would like to receive our non-technical preliminary project report when patient's test series is finished. Informant agreed to Test 4 at home, Tuesday, 9-15-64, at 10:30 a.m.

8-19-64. Patient called to let us know that she had changed her OPC appointment to Friday, 9-18-64.

8-20-64. Tried to contact patient by phone to let her know that we cannot co-ordinate our appointment for Test 4 with her OPC appointment. Patient not at home.

8-21-64. Called patient to schedule an appointment for Test 4. Explained to patient that we could not co-ordinate her 9-18-64 OPC visit with our research visit because of differences between OPC date and our research cycle dates. Suggested to patient that we see her at same time we see informant. Patient said that we would have to see her earlier because she had to leave for work at 11:00 a.m. Appointment for Test 4 for patient and informant on Tuesday, 9-15-64, at 10:00 a.m. at informant's home.

9-14-64. Mrs. King, informant, called and said she would not be able to keep appointment tomorrow because there has been a death in the family. A new appointment was scheduled for Thursday, 9-17-64, at 1:00 p.m. at home of informant.

9-17-64. Completed Test 4, informant only, at informant's home. Although patient's Test 4 was conducted at same time, the patient data should be filed with "Data Not to Be Used" as it had been 41 days (too long) since patient was last seen. Record Test 4, patient only, as "Missed." W.W.M. verified this decision. Next appointment: Test 5, patient and informant, at home, Thursday, 10-15-64, 1:30.

10-7-64. Patient called to ask about making an OPC appointment the day after our scheduled visit. I assured her that seeing her clinic doctor next day would not interfere with our plans for her or spoil our data. We will see her and informant as scheduled, 10-15-64.

10-15-64. Completed Test 5 as scheduled. Both informant and patient agreed to Test 6 at Mrs. King's (informant's) home on Monday, 11-16-64, at 1:30 p.m.

11-16-64. Patient and informant completed Test 6 as scheduled. Both agreed to Test 7 at Mrs. King's (informant's) home on Tuesday, 12-15-64, at 1:30 p.m.

11-19-64. Sent patient six-months letter of appreciation for taking part in study.

12-15-64. Patient and informant completed Test 7 as scheduled. Both agreed to Test 8 at informant's home on Thursday, 1-14-65, at 1:30 p.m.

1-14-65. Patient and informant completed Test 8 as scheduled. Both agreed to Test 9 at informant's home on Thursday, 2-11-65, at 1:30 p.m.

2-8-65. Called patient and changed appointment date for Test 9, because original appointment was inadvertently scheduled on a holiday. Patient agreed that she and informant would see us at informant's home on Thursday, 2-18-65, at 1:30 p.m. Patient said that she changed the appointment slip and her calendar notation while talking to me. A confirmation letter need *not* be sent in this case.

2-18-65. Patient and informant completed Test 9 at home as scheduled. Both agreed to Test 10 at informant's home on Thursday, 3-18-65, at 1:30 p.m.

3-15-65. Informant, Mrs. King, called the research office this morning. Said that in the past month it has been difficult living with the patient. The patient has been quick-tempered at home and at work; she has also avoided seeing people in the past two weeks. Mrs. King cancelled Test 10 because patient has a lawyer's appointment then. Mrs. King feels that patient should see her private physician immediately, but patient is presently unapproachable. I told informant that my schedule was free this afternoon; Test 10 was, therefore, rescheduled to Monday, 3-15-65, at 1:30 p.m.

3-15-65a. Patient and informant completed Test 10 at home as scheduled. Since our last contact (2-18-65) patient has had serious arguments with her employer, her husband and his lawyers, and her landlady-friend who is our informant. Informant, Mrs. King, was extremely upset in the interview. She said that the patient was defensive, argumentative, and erratic in behavior. In short, she has completely upset the routine of the house. Informant's account does not seem exaggerated. Patient will not consider any professional contact until Friday, 3-19-65. By this date a court case concerning visitation rights for patient and her son will have been held. I told both patient and informant that I would have a social worker contact them on Friday, 3-19-65, to help them work out their domestic situation. No definite appointment for Test 11 was set at this time; I said I would call back on Monday, 3-22-65, and arrange a Test 11 appointment.

3-15-65b. Visited social worker, Mrs. Alston, and related patient's problems to her. Mrs. Alston said that patient can best profit from her services if she is going to Spring Grove Outpatient Clinic, and promised to get in touch with her on Friday, 3-19-65.

3-16-65. Dora King (informant) called the research office this morning. She said that patient was somewhat improved after testing session 10 on 3-15-65; however, she does not know if she can permit the patient to continue living in her home. I suggested that she not make a hasty decision concerning the patient's living arrangement; that, in any event, she wait until Mrs. Alston (social worker) has contacted patient on Friday, 3-19-65. I also suggested that it was not inconceivable that the patient might spontaneously change for the better.

3-17-65. Dora King (informant) called the research office. She said that patient's activities yesterday evening were so disturbing to her (informant's) family that it is now necessary to have her rehospitalized. The most destructive of her activities was to call her employer on the phone, argue with her, and lose her job. She now has no significant source of income. I again stressed that informant should take no action until after the social worker, Mrs. Alston, has made her contact on 3-19-65. Mrs. King said she would call research office again on 3-18-65.

3-17-65a. Dora King (informant) called again this afternoon at 2:00. She said that several minutes ago patient was picked up at her home by police and was transported to Spring Grove. Mrs. King agreed to a relapse test, informant only, on Friday, 3-19-65, at 11:00 a.m. at her home.

3-17-65b. I left a note in Mrs. Alston's office that patient is now readmitted and should *not* be contacted.

3-18-65. Patient returned to Dayhoff Bldg., C Ward, ext. 404, on 3-17-65.

3-19-65. Informant only completed Relapse Test 11 as scheduled at her home. After testing, informant, who is patient's friend and landlady (Dora King), said that even if patient is released from hospital in time for Test 12, she does not expect to have contact with the patient and therefore cannot serve further as informant.

3-22-65. Called Dayhoff Building, C Ward, to schedule a relapse test for patient only. Patient has been moved to Sullivan Bldg., B Ward, ext. 231.

3-23-65. Called Sullivan Bldg., B Ward, ext. 231. Miss Jenkins, the nurse in charge, said that no research people are permitted in Sullivan Bldg. without the explicit approval of Dr. Stephens. Dr. Stephens is located in Dayhoff Bldg., and can be reached on ext. 408. I called Dr. Stephens, who approved my seeing patient for a relapse test. I then called Miss Jenkins a second time; it was agreed that patient be seen for a relapse test on Wednesday, 3-24-65, at 9:15 a.m.

3-24-65. Patient only completed relapse test on B Ward of Sullivan Bldg. as scheduled. As required by clinical policy in this building, nurse was in attendance throughout the entire testing session. This is Test 11, relapse test.

4-7-65. Checked hospital status of patient. Still in Sullivan Bldg., B Ward, ext. 231.

5-7-65. Checked hospital status of patient. Patient was transferred from Sullivan Bldg., B Ward, ext. 231, to Mitchell Bldg., B Ward, ext. 232, on 4-21-65.

5-7-65a. Patient is in hospital at Period 12; therefore no Test 12 will be given. Case Closed.

Appendix D

# *Record Form for Research Action Notes on Each Case

This form was used in each patient's research case file. Under "Action Taken," every staff-patient *transaction* was recorded in terse narrative style by the staff member involved. (*Data* were recorded and filed elsewhere.) The chronological entries were thus analogous to clinical notes: they provided a continuous and current record of the patient's research status. (A complete set of "Action Taken" notes on one case is exhibited in Appendix C.)

The two sections in the bottom half of the form were reserved for reminders of future test appointments, up-to-date addresses and telephone numbers for patient and informant, and any kind of exceptional or unaccustomed procedure needed for keeping research contact alive from month to month.

# APPENDIX D

Name: Last First Middle Initial — Case Number

Longitudinal Follow-Up Study – Form LS-7 – Actions Taken and Scheduled

| Date | By (Initials) | Action Taken |
| --- | --- | --- |
| | | Page ______ |

| Future Date | By (Initials) | Action Scheduled |
| --- | --- | --- |
| | | |

| Date | By (Initials) | Special Notes for Handling This Case |
| --- | --- | --- |
| | | |

Appendix E

# Katz Adjustment Scales: Patient Forms[1]

Monthly self-reports from patients were obtained on the forms reproduced in this appendix. The scales for informants follow in Appendix F. Each of the two pencil-and-paper questionnaires (patient's and informant's) comprises five subtests or "Forms." Four of these, Forms 2-5, are virtually identical in the two separate questionnaires. Form 1 deals with psychiatric symptoms in both questionnaires, but the patient reports on different symptoms from those in the informant instrument.

In this reproduction of the KAS we have omitted the face sheet (containing blanks for basic identifying information) and the notations for keypunching item responses for machine scoring. We have added, in parentheses, the title of each form. Minor revisions have recently been made in the scales and are not shown here.

[1]Reproduced (with modifications) by permission of authors and publisher, *Psychological Reports*, Southern Universities Press, Box 1441, Missoula, Montana 59801. Copies of the complete original monograph (Katz and Lyerly, 1963) are obtainable from the publisher.

APPENDIX E

KAS Form S1
(Symptom Discomfort)

| | Today or during the past few weeks | | | |
|---|---|---|---|---|
| | 1 | 2 | 3 | 4 |
| | have not had this complaint | bothers me a little | bothers me quite a bit | bothers me almost all the time |
| 1. Headaches | ____ | ____ | ____ | ____ |
| 2. Pains in the heart or chest | ____ | ____ | ____ | ____ |
| 3. Heart pounding or racing | ____ | ____ | ____ | ____ |
| 4. Trouble getting your breath | ____ | ____ | ____ | ____ |
| 5. Constipation | ____ | ____ | ____ | ____ |
| 6. Nausea, vomiting or upset stomach | ____ | ____ | ____ | ____ |
| 7. Loose bowel movements | ____ | ____ | ____ | ____ |
| 8. Twitching of the face or body | ____ | ____ | ____ | ____ |
| 9. Faintness or dizziness | ____ | ____ | ____ | ____ |
| 10. Hot or cold spells | ____ | ____ | ____ | ____ |
| 11. Itching | ____ | ____ | ____ | ____ |
| 12. Frequent urination | ____ | ____ | ____ | ____ |
| 13. Pains in the lower part of your back | ____ | ____ | ____ | ____ |
| 14. Difficulty in swallowing | ____ | ____ | ____ | ____ |
| 15. Skin eruptions or rashes | ____ | ____ | ____ | ____ |
| 16. Soreness of your muscles | ____ | ____ | ____ | ____ |
| 17. Nervousness and shakiness under pressure | ____ | ____ | ____ | ____ |

KAS Form S1 (continued)

| | Today or during the past few weeks | | | |
|---|---|---|---|---|
| | 1 | 2 | 3 | 4 |
| | have not had this complaint | bothers me a little | bothers me quite a bit | bothers me almost all the time |
| 18. Difficulty in falling asleep or staying asleep | ____ | ____ | ____ | ____ |
| 19. Sudden fright for no apparent reason | ____ | ____ | ____ | ____ |
| 20. Bad dreams | ____ | ____ | ____ | ____ |
| 21. Blaming yourself for things you did or failed to do | ____ | ____ | ____ | ____ |
| 22. Feeling generally worried or fretful | ____ | ____ | ____ | ____ |
| 23. Feeling blue | ____ | ____ | ____ | ____ |
| 24. Being easily moved to tears | ____ | ____ | ____ | ____ |
| 25. A need to do things very slowly in order to be sure you were doing them right | ____ | ____ | ____ | ____ |
| 26. Feeling like you have to do the same thing over and over again, like touching, counting, handwashing, etc. | ____ | ____ | ____ | ____ |
| 27. Unusual fears | ____ | ____ | ____ | ____ |
| 28. Thoughts or impulses which you don't like keep pushing themselves into your mind | ____ | ____ | ____ | ____ |
| 29. Your "feelings" being easily hurt | ____ | ____ | ____ | ____ |
| 30. Feeling that people were watching or talking about you | ____ | ____ | ____ | ____ |

KAS Form S1 (continued)

| | Today or during the past few weeks | | | |
|---|---|---|---|---|
| | 1 | 2 | 3 | 4 |
| | have not had this complaint | bothers me a little | bothers me quite a bit | bothers me almost all the time |
| 31. Preferring to be alone | ____ | ____ | ____ | ____ |
| 32. Feeling lonely | ____ | ____ | ____ | ____ |
| 33. Feeling like you have to ask others what you should do | ____ | ____ | ____ | ____ |
| 34. People being unsympathetic with your need for help | ____ | ____ | ____ | ____ |
| 35. Feeling easily annoyed or irritated | ____ | ____ | ____ | ____ |
| 36. Severe temper outbursts | ____ | ____ | ____ | ____ |
| 37. Feeling critical of others | ____ | ____ | ____ | ____ |
| 38. Frequently took medicine to make you feel better | ____ | ____ | ____ | ____ |
| 39. Difficulty in speaking when you were excited | ____ | ____ | ____ | ____ |
| 40. Feeling you were not functioning as well as you could, feeling blocked or unable to get things done | ____ | ____ | ____ | ____ |
| 41. Having an impulse to commit a violent or destructive act, for example, desire to set a fire, stab, beat or kill someone, mutilate an animal, etc. | ____ | ____ | ____ | ____ |
| 42. Blurring of vision | ____ | ____ | ____ | ____ |
| 43. Feeling thirsty | ____ | ____ | ____ | ____ |
| 44. Pains in arms or legs | ____ | ____ | ____ | ____ |

KAS Form S1 (continued)

| | Today or during the past few weeks | | | |
|---|---|---|---|---|
| | 1<br>have not had this complaint | 2<br>bothers me a little | 3<br>bothers me quite a bit | 4<br>bothers me almost all the time |
| 45. Loss of strength | ____ | ____ | ____ | ____ |
| 46. Dry mouth | ____ | ____ | ____ | ____ |
| 47. Pain in belly | ____ | ____ | ____ | ____ |
| 48. Feeling hungry | ____ | ____ | ____ | ____ |
| 49. Getting tired easily | ____ | ____ | ____ | ____ |
| 50. Feeling sleepy much of the time | ____ | ____ | ____ | ____ |
| 51. Keyed up and jittery | ____ | ____ | ____ | ____ |
| 52. Having no interest in things | ____ | ____ | ____ | ____ |
| 53. Having trouble keeping your mind on what you were doing | ____ | ____ | ____ | ____ |
| 54. Loss of appetite | ____ | ____ | ____ | ____ |
| 55. Having strange sexual ideas | ____ | ____ | ____ | ____ |

APPENDIX E

## KAS Form S2
(Level of Performance of Socially-Expected Activities)

| | 1<br>am not doing | 2<br>am doing some | 3<br>am doing regularly | 0<br>does not apply |
|---|---|---|---|---|
| 1. Help with household chores | ____ | ____ | ____ | ____ |
| 2. Visit friends | ____ | ____ | ____ | ____ |
| 3. Visit relatives | ____ | ____ | ____ | ____ |
| 4. Entertain friends at home | ____ | ____ | ____ | ____ |
| 5. Dress and take care of myself | ____ | ____ | ____ | ____ |
| 6. Help with the family budgeting | ____ | ____ | ____ | ____ |
| 7. Remember to do important things on time | ____ | ____ | ____ | ____ |
| 8. Get along with family members | ____ | ____ | ____ | ____ |
| 9. Go to parties and other social activites | ____ | ____ | ____ | ____ |
| 10. Get along with neighbors | ____ | ____ | ____ | ____ |
| 11. Help with family shopping | ____ | ____ | ____ | ____ |
| 12. Help in the care and training of children | ____ | ____ | ____ | ____ |
| 13. Go to church | ____ | ____ | ____ | ____ |
| 14. Take up hobbies | ____ | ____ | ____ | ____ |
| 15. Work | ____ | ____ | ____ | ____ |
| 16. Support the family | ____ | ____ | ____ | ____ |

APPENDIX E

KAS Form S3
(Level of Expectations)

| | 1<br>did not expect to be doing | 2<br>expected to be doing some | 3<br>expected to be doing regularly | 0<br>does not apply |
|---|---|---|---|---|
| 1. Help with household chores | ____ | ____ | ____ | ____ |
| 2. Visit friends | ____ | ____ | ____ | ____ |
| 3. Visit relatives | ____ | ____ | ____ | ____ |
| 4. Entertain friends at home | ____ | ____ | ____ | ____ |
| 5. Dress and take care of myself | ____ | ____ | ____ | ____ |
| 6. Help with the family budgeting | ____ | ____ | ____ | ____ |
| 7. Remember to do important things | ____ | ____ | ____ | ____ |
| 8. Get along with family members | ____ | ____ | ____ | ____ |
| 9. Go to parties and other social activities | ____ | ____ | ____ | ____ |
| 10. Get along with neighbors | ____ | ____ | ____ | ____ |
| 11. Help with family shopping | ____ | ____ | ____ | ____ |
| 12. Help in the care and training of children | ____ | ____ | ____ | ____ |
| 13. Go to church | ____ | ____ | ____ | ____ |
| 14. Take up hobbies | ____ | ____ | ____ | ____ |
| 15. Work | ____ | ____ | ____ | ____ |
| 16. Support the family | ____ | ____ | ____ | ____ |

APPENDIX E

## KAS Form RS4
(Level of Free-Time Activities)

| | 1<br>frequently | 2<br>some-<br>times | 3<br>practically<br>never | 0<br>does not<br>apply |
|---|---|---|---|---|
| 1. Work in and around the house | ____ | ____ | ____ | ____ |
| 2. Work in the garden or yard | ____ | ____ | ____ | ____ |
| 3. Work on some hobby | ____ | ____ | ____ | ____ |
| 4. Listen to the radio | ____ | ____ | ____ | ____ |
| 5. Watch television | ____ | ____ | ____ | ____ |
| 6. Write letters | ____ | ____ | ____ | ____ |
| 7. Go to the movies | ____ | ____ | ____ | ____ |
| 8. Attend lectures, theatre | ____ | ____ | ____ | ____ |
| 9. Attend club, lodge, other meetings | ____ | ____ | ____ | ____ |
| 10. Shop | ____ | ____ | ____ | ____ |
| 11. Take part in community or church work | ____ | ____ | ____ | ____ |
| 12. Bowl or other sports | ____ | ____ | ____ | ____ |
| 13. Play cards or other table games | ____ | ____ | ____ | ____ |
| 14. Take rides | ____ | ____ | ____ | ____ |
| 15. Visit friends | ____ | ____ | ____ | ____ |
| 16. Entertain friends | ____ | ____ | ____ | ____ |
| 17. Sew, crochet or knit | ____ | ____ | ____ | ____ |
| 18. Read | ____ | ____ | ____ | ____ |
| 19. Go to the library | ____ | ____ | ____ | ____ |
| 20. Just sit and think | ____ | ____ | ____ | ____ |
| 21. Take courses at home | ____ | ____ | ____ | ____ |
| 22. Go to school | ____ | ____ | ____ | ____ |
| 23. Other (what?) | ____ | ____ | ____ | ____ |

APPENDIX E

## KAS Form S5
(Level of Satisfaction with Free-Time Activities)

| | 1<br>satisfied with what I do here | 2<br>would like to do more of this | 3<br>would like to do less | 0<br>does not apply |
|---|---|---|---|---|
| 1. Work in and around the house | ____ | ____ | ____ | ____ |
| 2. Work in the garden or yard | ____ | ____ | ____ | ____ |
| 3. Work on some hobby | ____ | ____ | ____ | ____ |
| 4. Listen to the radio | ____ | ____ | ____ | ____ |
| 5. Watch television | ____ | ____ | ____ | ____ |
| 6. Write letters | ____ | ____ | ____ | ____ |
| 7. Go to the movies | ____ | ____ | ____ | ____ |
| 8. Attend lectures, theatre | ____ | ____ | ____ | ____ |
| 9. Attend club, lodge, other meetings | ____ | ____ | ____ | ____ |
| 10. Shop | ____ | ____ | ____ | ____ |
| 11. Take part in community or church work | ____ | ____ | ____ | ____ |
| 12. Bowl or other sports | ____ | ____ | ____ | ____ |
| 13. Play cards or other table games | ____ | ____ | ____ | ____ |
| 14. Take rides | ____ | ____ | ____ | ____ |
| 15. Visit friends | ____ | ____ | ____ | ____ |
| 16. Entertain friends | ____ | ____ | ____ | ____ |
| 17. Sew, crochet or knit | ____ | ____ | ____ | ____ |
| 18. Read | ____ | ____ | ____ | ____ |
| 19. Go to the library | ____ | ____ | ____ | ____ |
| 20. Just sit and think | ____ | ____ | ____ | ____ |
| 21. Take courses at home | ____ | ____ | ____ | ____ |
| 22. Go to school | ____ | ____ | ____ | ____ |
| 23. Other (what?) | ____ | ____ | ____ | ____ |

Appendix F

# Katz Adjustment Scales: Informant Forms[1]

See Appendix E for patient forms and for general information on the KAS.

---

KAS Form R1
(Relative's Ratings of Patient Symptoms and Social Behavior)

*Part I*

| | 1<br>almost never | 2<br>some-times | 3<br>often | 4<br>almost always |
|---|---|---|---|---|
| 1. Has trouble sleeping | ____ | ____ | ____ | ____ |
| 2. Gets very self-critical, starts to blame himself for things | ____ | ____ | ____ | ____ |
| 3. Cries easily | ____ | ____ | ____ | ____ |
| 4. Feels lonely | ____ | ____ | ____ | ____ |
| 5. Acts as if he has no interest in things | ____ | ____ | ____ | ____ |
| 6. Is restless | ____ | ____ | ____ | ____ |

[1] Reproduced by permission: See Appendix E, footnote 1.

KAS Form R1 (continued)

| | 1<br>almost never | 2<br>some-times | 3<br>often | 4<br>almost always |
|---|---|---|---|---|
| 7. Has periods where he can't stop moving or doing something | ____ | ____ | ____ | ____ |
| 8. Just sits | ____ | ____ | ____ | ____ |
| 9. Acts as if he doesn't have much energy | ____ | ____ | ____ | ____ |
| 10. Looks worn out | ____ | ____ | ____ | ____ |
| 11. Feelings get hurt easily | ____ | ____ | ____ | ____ |
| 12. Feels that people don't care about him | ____ | ____ | ____ | ____ |
| 13. Does the same thing over and over again without reason | ____ | ____ | ____ | ____ |
| 14. Passes out | ____ | ____ | ____ | ____ |
| 15. Gets very sad, blue | ____ | ____ | ____ | ____ |
| 16. Tries too hard | ____ | ____ | ____ | ____ |
| 17. Needs to do things very slowly to do them right | ____ | ____ | ____ | ____ |
| 18. Has strange fears | ____ | ____ | ____ | ____ |
| 19. Afraid something terrible is going to happen | ____ | ____ | ____ | ____ |
| 20. Gets nervous easily | ____ | ____ | ____ | ____ |
| 21. Jittery | ____ | ____ | ____ | ____ |
| 22. Worries or frets | ____ | ____ | ____ | ____ |
| 23. Gets sudden fright for no reason | ____ | ____ | ____ | ____ |
| 24. Has bad dreams | ____ | ____ | ____ | ____ |
| 25. Acts as if he sees people or things that aren't there | ____ | ____ | ____ | ____ |
| 26. Does strange things without reason | ____ | ____ | ____ | ____ |

KAS Form R1 (continued)

| | 1 almost never | 2 some-times | 3 often | 4 almost always |
|---|---|---|---|---|
| 27. Attempts suicide | ____ | ____ | ____ | ____ |
| 28. Gets angry and breaks things | ____ | ____ | ____ | ____ |
| 29. Talks to himself | ____ | ____ | ____ | ____ |
| 30. Acts as if he has no control over his emotions | ____ | ____ | ____ | ____ |
| 31. Laughs or cries at strange times | ____ | ____ | ____ | ____ |
| 32. Has mood changes without reason | ____ | ____ | ____ | ____ |
| 33. Has temper tantrums | ____ | ____ | ____ | ____ |
| 34. Gets very excited for no reason | ____ | ____ | ____ | ____ |
| 35. Gets very happy for no reason | ____ | ____ | ____ | ____ |
| 36. Acts as if he doesn't care about other people's feelings | ____ | ____ | ____ | ____ |
| 37. Thinks only of himself | ____ | ____ | ____ | ____ |
| 38. Shows his feelings | ____ | ____ | ____ | ____ |
| 39. Generous | ____ | ____ | ____ | ____ |
| 40. Thinks people are talking about him | ____ | ____ | ____ | ____ |
| 41. Complains of headaches, stomach trouble, other physical ailments | ____ | ____ | ____ | ____ |
| 42. Bossy | ____ | ____ | ____ | ____ |
| 43. Acts as if he's suspicious of people | ____ | ____ | ____ | ____ |
| 44. Argues | ____ | ____ | ____ | ____ |
| 45. Gets into fights with people | ____ | ____ | ____ | ____ |
| 46. Is cooperative | ____ | ____ | ____ | ____ |

KAS Form R1 (continued)

| | 1<br>almost never | 2<br>some-times | 3<br>often | 4<br>almost always |
|---|---|---|---|---|
| 47. Does the opposite of what he is asked | ____ | ____ | ____ | ____ |
| 48. Stubborn | ____ | ____ | ____ | ____ |
| 49. Answers when talked to | ____ | ____ | ____ | ____ |
| 50. Curses at people | ____ | ____ | ____ | ____ |
| 51. Deliberately upsets routine | ____ | ____ | ____ | ____ |
| 52. Resentful | ____ | ____ | ____ | ____ |
| 53. Envious of other people | ____ | ____ | ____ | ____ |
| 54. Friendly | ____ | ____ | ____ | ____ |
| 55. Gets annoyed easily | ____ | ____ | ____ | ____ |
| 56. Critical of other people | ____ | ____ | ____ | ____ |
| 57. Pleasant | ____ | ____ | ____ | ____ |
| 58. Gets along well with people | ____ | ____ | ____ | ____ |
| 59. Lies | ____ | ____ | ____ | ____ |
| 60. Gets into trouble with law | ____ | ____ | ____ | ____ |
| 61. Gets drunk | ____ | ____ | ____ | ____ |
| 62. Is dependable | ____ | ____ | ____ | ____ |
| 63. Is responsible | ____ | ____ | ____ | ____ |
| 64. Doesn't argue (talk) back | ____ | ____ | ____ | ____ |
| 65. Obedient | ____ | ____ | ____ | ____ |
| 66. Shows good judgment | ____ | ____ | ____ | ____ |
| 67. Stays away from people | ____ | ____ | ____ | ____ |
| 68. Takes drugs other than recommended by hospital or clinic | ____ | ____ | ____ | ____ |
| 69. Shy | ____ | ____ | ____ | ____ |
| 70. Quiet | ____ | ____ | ____ | ____ |
| 71. Prefers to be alone | ____ | ____ | ____ | ____ |

## KAS Form R1 (continued)

| | 1<br>almost never | 2<br>some-times | 3<br>often | 4<br>almost always |
|---|---|---|---|---|
| 72. Needs a lot of attention | ____ | ____ | ____ | ____ |
| 73. Behavior is childish | ____ | ____ | ____ | ____ |
| 74. Acts helpless | ____ | ____ | ____ | ____ |
| 75. Is independent | ____ | ____ | ____ | ____ |

*Part II*

| | | | | |
|---|---|---|---|---|
| 1. Moves about very slowly | ____ | ____ | ____ | ____ |
| 2. Moves about in a hurried way | ____ | ____ | ____ | ____ |
| 3. Clumsy; keeps bumping into things or dropping things | ____ | ____ | ____ | ____ |
| 4. Very quick to react to something you say or do | ____ | ____ | ____ | ____ |
| 5. Very slow to react | ____ | ____ | ____ | ____ |
| 6. Gets into peculiar positions | ____ | ____ | ____ | ____ |
| 7. Makes peculiar movements | ____ | ____ | ____ | ____ |
| 8. Hands tremble | ____ | ____ | ____ | ____ |
| 9. Will stay in one position for a long period | ____ | ____ | ____ | ____ |
| 10. Loses track of day, month, or year | ____ | ____ | ____ | ____ |
| 11. Forgets his address or other places he knows well | ____ | ____ | ____ | ____ |
| 12. Remembers the names of people he knows well | ____ | ____ | ____ | ____ |
| 13. Acts as if he doesn't know where he is | ____ | ____ | ____ | ____ |

KAS Form R1 (continued)

| | 1<br>almost never | 2<br>some-times | 3<br>often | 4<br>almost always |
|---|---|---|---|---|
| 14. Remembers important things | ____ | ____ | ____ | ____ |
| 15. Acts as if he's confused about things; in a daze | ____ | ____ | ____ | ____ |
| 16. Acts as if he can't get certain thoughts out of his mind | ____ | ____ | ____ | ____ |
| 17. Acts as if he can't concentrate on one thing | ____ | ____ | ____ | ____ |
| 18. Acts as if he can't make decisions | ____ | ____ | ____ | ____ |
| 19. Talks without making sense | ____ | ____ | ____ | ____ |
| 20. Hard to understand his words | ____ | ____ | ____ | ____ |
| 21. Speaks clearly | ____ | ____ | ____ | ____ |
| 22. Refuses to speak at all for periods of time | ____ | ____ | ____ | ____ |
| 23. Speaks so low you cannot hear him | ____ | ____ | ____ | ____ |
| 24. Speaks very loudly | ____ | ____ | ____ | ____ |
| 25. Shouts or yells for no reason | ____ | ____ | ____ | ____ |
| 26. Speaks very fast | ____ | ____ | ____ | ____ |
| 27. Speaks very slowly | ____ | ____ | ____ | ____ |
| 28. Acts as if he wants to speak but can't | ____ | ____ | ____ | ____ |
| 29. Keeps repeating the same idea | ____ | ____ | ____ | ____ |
| 30. Keeps changing from one subject to another for no reason | ____ | ____ | ____ | ____ |

KAS Form R1 (continued)

| | 1<br>almost never | 2<br>some-times | 3<br>often | 4<br>almost always |
|---|---|---|---|---|
| 31. Talks too much | ____ | ____ | ____ | ____ |
| 32. Says that people are talking about him | ____ | ____ | ____ | ____ |
| 33. Says that people are trying to make him do or think things he doesn't want to | ____ | ____ | ____ | ____ |
| 34. Talks as if he committed the worst sins | ____ | ____ | ____ | ____ |
| 35. Talks about how angry he is at certain people | ____ | ____ | ____ | ____ |
| 36. Talks about people or things he's very afraid of | ____ | ____ | ____ | ____ |
| 37. Threatens to injure certain people | ____ | ____ | ____ | ____ |
| 38. Threatens to tell people off | ____ | ____ | ____ | ____ |
| 39. Says he is afraid that he will injure somebody | ____ | ____ | ____ | ____ |
| 40. Says he is afraid that he will not be able to control himself | ____ | ____ | ____ | ____ |
| 41. Talks about strange things that are going on inside his body | ____ | ____ | ____ | ____ |
| 42. Says how bad or useless he is | ____ | ____ | ____ | ____ |
| 43. Brags about how good he is | ____ | ____ | ____ | ____ |
| 44. Says the same thing over and over again | ____ | ____ | ____ | ____ |

## KAS Form R1 (continued)

| | 1<br>almost never | 2<br>some-times | 3<br>often | 4<br>almost always |
|---|---|---|---|---|
| 45. Complains about people and things in general | ____ | ____ | ____ | ____ |
| 46. Talks about big plans he has for the future | ____ | ____ | ____ | ____ |
| 47. Says or acts as if people are after him | ____ | ____ | ____ | ____ |
| 48. Says that something terrible is going to happen | ____ | ____ | ____ | ____ |
| 49. Believes in strange things | ____ | ____ | ____ | ____ |
| 50. Talks about suicide | ____ | ____ | ____ | ____ |
| 51. Talks about strange sexual ideas | ____ | ____ | ____ | ____ |
| 52. Gives advice without being asked | ____ | ____ | ____ | ____ |

# APPENDIX F

## KAS Form R2
(Level of Performance of Socially-Expected Activities)

| | 1<br>is not doing | 2<br>is doing some | 3<br>is doing regularly | 0<br>does not apply |
|---|---|---|---|---|
| 1. Helps with household chores | _____ | _____ | _____ | _____ |
| 2. Visits his friends | _____ | _____ | _____ | _____ |
| 3. Visits his relatives | _____ | _____ | _____ | _____ |
| 4. Entertains friends at home | _____ | _____ | _____ | _____ |
| 5. Dresses and takes care of himself | _____ | _____ | _____ | _____ |
| 6. Helps with the family budgeting | _____ | _____ | _____ | _____ |
| 7. Remembers to do important things on time | _____ | _____ | _____ | _____ |
| 8. Gets along with family members | _____ | _____ | _____ | _____ |
| 9. Goes to parties and other social activities | _____ | _____ | _____ | _____ |
| 10. Gets along with neighbors | _____ | _____ | _____ | _____ |
| 11. Helps with family shopping | _____ | _____ | _____ | _____ |
| 12. Helps in the care and training of children | _____ | _____ | _____ | _____ |
| 13. Goes to church | _____ | _____ | _____ | _____ |
| 14. Takes up hobbies | _____ | _____ | _____ | _____ |
| 15. Works | _____ | _____ | _____ | _____ |
| 16. Supports the family | _____ | _____ | _____ | _____ |

APPENDIX F

## KAS Form R3
(Level of Expectations)

| | 1<br>did not expect him to be doing | 2<br>expected him to be doing some | 3<br>expected him to be doing regularly | 0<br>does not apply |
|---|---|---|---|---|
| 1. Helps with household chores | ____ | ____ | ____ | ____ |
| 2. Visits his friends | ____ | ____ | ____ | ____ |
| 3. Visits his relatives | ____ | ____ | ____ | ____ |
| 4. Entertains friends at home | ____ | ____ | ____ | ____ |
| 5. Dresses and takes care of himself | ____ | ____ | ____ | ____ |
| 6. Helps with the family budgeting | ____ | ____ | ____ | ____ |
| 7. Remembers to do important things on time | ____ | ____ | ____ | ____ |
| 8. Gets along with family members | ____ | ____ | ____ | ____ |
| 9. Goes to parties and other social activities | ____ | ____ | ____ | ____ |
| 10. Gets along with neighbors | ____ | ____ | ____ | ____ |
| 11. Helps with family shopping | ____ | ____ | ____ | ____ |
| 12. Helps in the care and training of children | ____ | ____ | ____ | ____ |
| 13. Goes to church | ____ | ____ | ____ | ____ |
| 14. Takes up hobbies | ____ | ____ | ____ | ____ |
| 15. Works | ____ | ____ | ____ | ____ |
| 16. Supports the family | ____ | ____ | ____ | ____ |

## APPENDIX F

# KAS Forms RS4, R5

[These two informant forms are exactly the same as the last two patient forms, Appendix E, except that in Form R5 the column headings read:

1 satisfied with what he does here

2 would like to see him do more of this

3 would like to see him do less

0 does not apply]

Appendix G

# *Supplemental Instructions for the Administration of the Katz Adjustment Scales

Our project was among the first in which the Katz Adjustment Scales were used extensively. This manual was prepared in order to resolve technical problems with the KAS that had arisen early in the course of data collection. Its immediate purpose was to standardize our own procedure and to help train our Examiners. It was intended also as an aid for other users of the KAS.

The manual was written by Kathleen H. Gansereit, William W. Michaux, Martin M. Katz, and Henri A. Lowery.

---

Basic instructions for administering the Katz Adjustment Scales (KAS) have been presented elsewhere (Katz and Lyerly, 1963, pp. 533-535). The addenda in this manual were developed out of extensive experience with the scales in research on patients newly discharged from a mental hospital. It has proved advisable to provide these additional rules of thumb for the examiner so as to minimize errors of measurement. Some of these rules apply to the testing procedure in general, others to specific subtests (Forms), items, or response options.

## INDEPENDENT TESTING OF PATIENT AND INFORMANT

When administering both the R Forms and the S Forms at a single session, make sure that the patient and informant (usually a relative of the patient) are not within earshot of each other at any time from the start of the first test to the completion of the second. Independent tests are imperative to ensure validity. When tests are done on home visits, i.e., when the examiner goes to the home of the patient and/or relative to administer the KAS to both parties, privacy for separate tests is occasionally difficult to arrange. Be tactful but firm in making certain there is no communication, either intentional or inadvertent, between patient and relative during testing.

## EXPLAINING THE DIRECTIONS

Suggested wordings for starting the patient and relative on each subtest are given in the basic KAS instructions. Whenever a subject has difficulty in understanding these oral directions, it is entirely permissible to rephrase or explain them, provided the original meaning is kept. It is also permissible to read the entire test aloud to any subject who has serious limitations of eyesight, literacy, or verbal comprehension. In such cases, repeat the response choices occasionally to be sure the subject has them clearly in mind. The examiner may also mark the answers as reported orally by the subject, whenever this seems preferable to having the subject mark them.

## EXAMINER'S PRESENCE ESSENTIAL

The examiner must be on hand throughout testing—though not necessarily in the subject's immediate presence at all times. He may, for example, start the relative on Form R1, then start the patient on the S Forms in another room, and thereafter divide his time between the two. Under no circumstances should the KAS forms be left with a subject to complete on his own. The examiner must remain present not only to give the instructions for each subtest, but also to monitor the test. Monitoring is covered in the remainder of this manual.

## MONITORING THE TESTS

### *Erratic Response Patterns*

Careful but unobtrusive monitoring of test-taking is essential, though the amount of active intervention needed varies greatly from one subject to another. Obviously many subjects who take the S Forms will be disturbed persons; this will sometimes be manifested in erratic test-taking behavior, and occasionally relatives will also display such behavior. The two most common erratic response patterns are skipping items and position preference, i.e. marking all responses in the same column. It is desirable to spot and correct such tendencies early in the session before they become entrenched.

*Emotional Resistance*

Some patients and relatives display mild emotional resistance to testing by tending to gloss over symptomatic behavior or by quibbling over response choices. A common form of resistance is "discounting": a subject readily admits a symptom, but then tries to explain it away circumstantially and proposes not to mark it as present. Somatic complaints are prime targets for discounting. In such instances, press for a straightforward factual report of all that has happened in the period being covered, explaining if need be that personal judgments cannot fairly be incorporated into the test responses.

In some few highly suspicious subjects, usually patients, a more severe form of resistance is encountered: The KAS is seen as a device for gathering damning evidence. Whenever this kind of antipathy is expressed, it behooves the examiner to explain openly and honestly, in so far as allowable in his working context, the nature and purpose of the KAS. Moreover, even when this kind of distrust is not divulged, the examiner can often facilitate rapport by taking the initiative in telling the subject just what the test is for. Occasional testing failures must still be expected, but this approach will do much to enhance cooperativeness and KAS validity.

*Helping with Specific Responses*

Within these limits, the patient and the relative should be allowed to make their own choices of responses to mark, even though some answers may seem inaccurate to the examiner. In making their choices, however, they will sometimes need help in understanding just what is called for. The alert examiner will detect these trouble spots and discuss them with the subject to provide clarification and guidance. The general rule for helping with any particular item is: Explain freely the meaning of anything in the KAS booklets (carefully avoiding compromise or distortion), but never direct or wheedle the subject as he judges which response choice is most appropriate in his case. In short, serve as a glossary but not as an arbitrator. The rule may need modification in some instances; see below.

### *Form R1: Relative's Ratings of Patient Symptoms and Social Behavior*

The relative should answer *all items*, each according to his own judgment. For items on which he lacks adequate information about the patient and is unsure of the appropriate response, he should be told to mark column 1, "almost never." This means simply that, *so far as the relative knows*, the behavior in question has not recently occurred to any significant degree. In other instances in Form R1, the relative may object to marking "almost never" on the grounds that he knows the correct response is really "never." If this happens, explain that "almost never" includes the notion of "never" and is so counted in scoring and interpreting. In monitoring Form R1, make sure the relative sees that not all of the items describe abnormal or undesirable behavior. The most clear-cut exceptions are items 39, 46, 49, 54, 57, 58, 62, 63, 66, 75, 87 (12), 89 (14), and 96 (21). (Numbers in parentheses are alternate item numbers: in some versions of the KAS, Form R1 is divided into two parts, so that item 87 becomes item 12 of Part II, and so on.)

### *Forms R3 and S3: Level of Expectations*

The task of retrospectively reporting one's expectations in Forms R3 and S3 is somewhat more complex than the kind of current factual report called for in all the other forms. It becomes still more complex if the KAS is given repeatedly to the same subjects, e.g., in a longitudinal study. In such cases, for each successive test the retrospective reference-point for expectations will ordinarily remain the same–viz., the time when the patient was discharged. On the other hand, the current period against which the expectations are repeatedly measured will change from test to test. At each consecutive testing, the subject can be asked to report to what extent the various activities were expected to be engaged in "at this time." Make sure the subject knows what is being asked for, but do not belabor the notion of retrospective report. As Katz and Lyerly state in the monograph cited above, "It is not necessary to assume that the retrospective level is an accurate estimate of the relative's expectations at discharge. . . . The intention is to measure his present perception of that previous level" (Katz and Lyerly, 1963, p. 515, footnote 4). The same point applies to the patient's report of his own self-expectations in Form S3.

### *Form RS4: Level of Free-Time Activities*

Some subjects have difficulty in drawing the line between "frequently" and "sometimes," or between "sometimes" and "practically never." Use the following for clarification if needed:

"Frequently" means: "very often, a lot, fairly regularly"

"Sometimes" means: "once in a while" (but *not*: "once only")

"Practically never" means: either "once only" or "never."

Item 23, "Other (what?)," is a write-in item to be used only if the subject wishes to add a free-time activity which he feels is important. Most subjects leave this item blank unless it is called to their attention. Skipping this item is permissible; it is not ordinarily scored. The same applies to the corresponding write-in item No. 23 in Forms R5 and S5.

### *Form S1: Symptom Discomfort*

In Form S1 the item most likely to puzzle patients is No. 38, "Frequently took medicine to make you feel better." If difficulty arises here, first ascertain whether medicine *has* been used. If it has not, the proper response will always be "1: have not had this complaint." For patients who do take medicine, the item can be paraphrased: "To what degree does it bother you that you must take medicine?" and the patient can respond accordingly.

### *The "Does Not Apply" Response*

This response option is found in all KAS Forms except the R1 and S1. Discourage any patient or relative from using it too freely. Allow its use only after making sure the individual situation justifies it for any particular item. For example, a housewife who has no children might reasonably answer "does not apply" to item 12 in Form S2, "*Help*(s) in the care and training of children." Even here, however, the item *would* apply to a childless woman if she were living in a community or family setting where it was commonly socially expected for women to help in caring for other people's children. Among the items which frequently come under fire for the "does not apply" response are:

In Forms R2, S2, R3, and S3:

3. Visit(s) (his) relatives
6. Help(s) with the family budgeting
10. Get(s) along with neighbors
11. Help(s) with family shopping
15. Work(s)
16. Support(s) the family

In Forms RS4, R5, and S5:

2. Work in the garden or yard
17. Sew, crochet, or knit (Construe this item as applicable to males as well as to females)
21. Take courses at home
22. Go to school

The general rule is: The "does not apply" response is acceptable only when: (1) the patient's social role leaves the activity unequivocally out of the question, or (2) the environment makes it physically impossible for the patient to perform a given activity. Examples: (1) Social role: an unmarried patient living alone could mark "does not apply" for "help with the family budgeting." (2) Environment: a patient living on the tenth floor of a downtown apartment building could mark "does not apply" for "work in the garden or yard." In the two following examples, on the other hand, the "does not apply" response should *not* be allowed: (1) Social role: "Support the family" *does* apply to a married woman despite her saying that "My husband supports the family, and I have three small children to care for at home." (Husbands can become incapacitated or improvident.) (2) Environment: "Visit relatives" *does* apply even when a patient says "my nearest relatives live 150 miles from here." (Out-of-town visits are not impossible.)

## ENSURING THAT THE TEST IS COMPLETE

Encouraging subjects to answer all items will help to ensure complete protocols, but will not forestall occasional lapses. Inadvertent skipping can happen not only for a single item but also for a whole page or form. Before dismissing any subject, always check the entire KAS booklet for missing responses. If despite this precaution missing responses are found later, do not complete them, even though you may be confident you have the correct information. The KAS can be adequately scored even when a few items are left incomplete.

*Reference:* Katz, M. M., and Lyerly, S. B. Methods for measuring adjustment and social behavior in the community: I. Rationale, description, discriminative validity and scale development. *Psychol. Rep.*, 1963, 13, 503-535.

Appendix H

# *Life-Situation Interview: Patient Form

For the monthly sessions with patients, each evaluation comprised, in addition to the Katz Adjustment Scales (Patient Forms), 27 interview items used by the Examiner. Fourteen of the interview items (5 to 7 and 17 to 27) had virtually identical counterparts in the informant interview form presented in Appendix I. The remaining 13 items (1 to 4 and 8 to 16) were used only in the patient interview.

In this reproduction of our original interview form we have eliminated all non-substantive material such as record-keeping items and cues for coding and keypunching. We have also undertaken to improve the original wording at a few points. The categorical structure of the data as collected in the interview has not been altered, however.

---

*I. Outpatient Treatment*

1. Main source of outpatient psychiatric treatment during current period:
   None
   Spring Grove Outpatient Clinic
   Other public clinic: ____________________
   City
   Private psychiatrist

Private physician
Visiting Public Health Nurse
Other (Specify): ____________________

2. Secondary source of outpatient psychiatric treatment during current period:
(Same answers as for item 1)

3. Other source(s) of outpatient psychiatric treatment during current period:
None
Other source(s) (Specify): ____________________

4. Current and anticipated status of outpatient psychiatric treatment:
None currently received or planned
None now, but definitely planning to start soon
Received during current period, but stopped as of last visit
Receiving now, but definitely plans to stop soon
Receiving now, plans to continue

5. During current period, how much of time has patient had psychiatric drug(s) *prescribed*? (Disregard actual consumption in this item. If patient failed to refill prescription as instructed, count as time *on* prescribed drug.)
None of the time during current period
Less than half of the time
About half of the time
More than half of the time
All of the time

Name of drug(s):

____________________

6. According to patient's report, how long has he *used* above psychiatric drug(s) throughout total time *prescribed* during current period?
No use of prescribed drug(s)
Less than half of the time prescribed
About half of the time prescribed
More than half of the time prescribed
All of the time prescribed
Longer than the time prescribed
Not applicable: no drug prescribed

7. According to patient's report, to what extent has his typical daily use of psychiatric drug(s) during current period adhered to the prescribed dosage?
   No use of prescribed drug(s)
   Less than half of prescribed daily dosage
   About half of prescribed daily dosage
   More than half of prescribed daily dosage
   Equal to prescribed daily dosage
   More than prescribed daily dosage
   Not applicable: no drug prescribed

8. Has patient received any *outpatient* psychiatric treatment *other than* drugs during current period?
   Yes (Check one or more):
      Individual psychotherapy
      Group psychotherapy
      Public Health Nurse Visit(s), not limited to providing drugs
      Electroshock
      Other (Specify): ____________________
   No

*II. Home and Family*

9. Type of home in which patient now lives:
   Marital
   Parental
   Other relative(s)
   Common-law
   Alone
   Other (Specify): ____________________

10. Number of own children *living with patient* __________

11. Number of stepchildren or in-law children *living with patient* __________

12. Number of own children living *apart from patient* __________

13. Present marital status:
    Single
    Married
    Divorced
    Separated
    Widowed

14. Closest living relative:
    No known living blood relative or spouse
    Spouse
    Parent
    Son and/or daughter
    Sibling
    Uncle and/or aunt
    Other (Specify):____________________

15. Is mother living?
    Yes
    No
    Uncertain

16. Is father living?
    Yes
    No
    Uncertain

*III. Homemaking and Work*

17. Female patients: present functioning as homemaker:
    Sole responsibility as homemaker
    Shares responsibility as homemaker
    Maintains home, but only for self
    No responsibility as homemaker
    Not applicable: male patient

18. How much of the time has patient been gainfully employed during current period?
    None of the time during current period
    Less than half of the time
    About half of the time
    More than half of the time
    All of the time

19. What is the highest number of hours patient has worked in a single week during current period?
    1 to 17 hours in a week
    18 to 34 hours in a week
    35 or more hours in a week
    Not applicable: unemployed for entire period

*IV. Recent and Current Life Stresses*

20 to 27. (The eight environmental stress questions which terminated the patient interview are presented separately in Appendix J. Compared with the rest of the interview items, they are clinically more sensitive and psychometrically less simple. Appendix J provides the necessary explanation.)

Appendix I

# *Life – Situation Interview: Informant Form

For the monthly sessions with informants, each evaluation comprised, in addition to the Katz Adjustment Scales (Informant Forms), 16 interview items used by the examiner. Except for numbers 7 and 16, all of the items had virtually identical counterparts in the patient interview form presented in Appendix H. In the following reproduction of our original informant interview form we have made the same kinds of minor changes as noted for the patient form.

---

*I. Drug Treatment*

1. During current period, how much of time has patient had psychiatric drug(s) *prescribed*? (Disregard actual consumption in this item. If patient failed to refill prescription as instructed, count as time *on* prescribed drug.)
   None of the time during current period
   Less than half of the time
   About half of the time — Name of drug(s):
   More than half of the time
   All of the time — ________________
   Informant does not know

2. According to informant's report, how long has patient *used* above psychiatric drug(s) throughout total time *prescribed* during current period?
   No use of prescribed drug(s)
   Less than half of the time prescribed
   About half of the time prescribed
   More than half of the time prescribed
   All of the time prescribed
   Longer than the time prescribed
   Informant does not know
   Not applicable: no drug prescribed

3. According to informant's report, to what extent has patient's typical daily use of psychiatric drug(s) during current period adhered to the prescribed dosage?
   No use of prescribed drug(s)
   Less than half of prescribed daily dosage
   About half of prescribed daily dosage
   More than half of prescribed daily dosage
   Equal to prescribed daily dosage
   More than prescribed daily dosage
   Informant does not know
   Not applicable: no drug prescribed

*II. Homemaking and Work*

4. Female patients: present functioning as homemaker:
   Sole responsibility as homemaker
   Shares responsibility as homemaker
   Maintains home, but only for self
   No responsibility as homemaker
   Informant does not know
   Not applicable: male patient

5. According to informant's report, how much of the time has patient been gainfully employed during current period?
   None of the time during current period
   Less than half of the time
   About half of the time
   More than half of the time
   All of the time
   Informant does not know

6. According to informant's report, what is the highest number of hours patient has worked in a single week during current period?
   1 to 17 hours in a week
   18 to 24 hours in a week
   35 or more hours in a week
   Informant does not know
   Not applicable: unemployed for entire period

7. To what extent is patient now contributing to financial support of his or her family?
   Sole breadwinner
   Major breadwinner
   Shares breadwinning about equally with other(s)
   Minor function as breadwinner
   Does not contribute to support of family
   Not applicable: no dependents to support

*III. Recent and Current Life Stresses*

8 to 15. (The eight environmental stress questions are presented separately in Appendix J. Compared with the rest of the interview items, they are clinically more sensitive and psychometrically less simple. Appendix J provides the necessary explanation.)

*IV. Source of Information*

16. Informant's relationship to patient:
    Spouse
    Mother
    Father
    Son
    Daughter
    Brother
    Sister
    Other, male (Specify): ____________________
    Other, female (Specify): ____________________

Appendix J

# Interview Inquiry into Recent and Current Life Stresses[1]

The eight items in our environmental stress inquiry were part of the life situation interview with both the patient and his informant (Appendixes H and I). Except for necessary changes in personal pronouns, the items were worded the same for both respondents; it is the patient form which is presented below.

Each stress question calls for a "yes" or "no" answer. In our own study, where the items were first used, examiners also recorded, for the first two items only, respondents' descriptions of the actual events signified by all "yes" answers. (We used this material in training examiners and standardizing interview procedure, and are retaining it for further work on refining the stress inquiry.) Examiners also found it desirable, when completing items 3 to 8, to note down the details of any "yes" answer which they could not immediately classify as to specific area of stress; they could thus avoid snap-judgment error and could complete the six-choice area coding without distraction after the interview was finished.

The first two items in the stress inquiry are auxiliary to, and separate from, the remaining six; they were designed partly as buffer questions, to provide easy transition from the earlier, less

[1]Reproduced (with modifications) by permission of the *Community Mental Health J.* from Michaux, Gansereit, McCabe, and Kurland, 1967. 3: 358-72.

personal part of our interview and to introduce the notion of stress as a subject of discussion. For identification, we call items 1 plus 2 the "General Stress Index." It is possible to score them additively as a three-point "scale" ranging from 0 to 2–viz.:

| | Score: | |
|---|---|---|
| Item | Yes | No |
| 1 | 0 | 1 |
| 2 | 1 | 0 |

Item 1, as seen by its content below, deals with the converse of stress; hence it is scored in the opposite direction to item 2–on the premise that the lack of any memorably favorable experiences during a 30-day period is in itself a form of stress and that, on the other hand, if such experiences *have* occurred, they would tend to mitigate the impact of any stress reported in item 2. Thus, despite the narrow range of possible total scores from 0 to 2, the General Stress Index does contain a "correction factor" which is lacking in the main inquiry.

Items 3-8 constitute the main inquiry, titled the Specific Stress Index. In these questions, the examiner's approach becomes more structured as he defines not only stress but also the six areas of patient experience in which he is interested. The area definitions serve also as cues to the respondent, suggesting material he might otherwise not report. The six areas are meant to include all possible contexts of experience which an adult subject might perceive as stressful or threatening.

Each specific stress item is scored 1 for "yes" and 0 for "no." The total score is the number of "yes" answers. During the interview, the respondent must document each "yes" answer in order for the interviewer to evaluate and classify the response–that is, decide whether it is a genuine yes, and if so, which of the six areas it belongs in.

Psychometrically, the apparent simplicity and straight forwardness of the specific stress index are deceptive: Excessive error of measurement is a distinct hazard both in the yes-or-no option and in the choice of area. While the interviewer's evaluation and recording of any response may agree with the respondent's original formulation of it, this is by no means always the case. In other words, affirmative answers cannot be taken at face value. We adopted three standards for acceptable "yes" answers on the specific stress index:

*1. Phenomenology:* Whether or not personal stress from a given episode would be normally expected is beside the point; adhere to the *patient's own phenomenology*—even, for example, if delusional material is inseparable from his perception of an event as stressful.

*2. Environment:* There must be a specifiable *external factor* in the form of some force, action, or development originating outside the patient, in his social or physical environment.

*3. Distress:* There must also be a clear-cut *subjective factor* in the form of distress, anxiety, or the like on the part of the patient—not necessarily hopelessness or panic, but something more than a mild or passing concern.

To clarify points 2 and 3, the interviewer must often improvise a few accessory questions to follow the standard ones. In our experience, vigilant observance of these rules is imperative, especially in view of the brevity and restricted range of the specific stress index. Moreover, these rules alone are not enough. If the reader should use the technique in other work, he will rather frequently encounter responses that require special interpretive decisions. In the interest of reliable measurement, it is essential for such decisions to be consistent from item to item. In our own work we ensured consistency by holding periodic staff meetings to discuss these (along with other) problems. For each interpretive problem, a staff consensus was reached and was thenceforth followed for responses posing the same problem.

---

1. "During the past month, has anything *very good* happened in your life—something that made you very happy or helped you to feel a lot better?"

   ____Yes (Specify): ______________________________
   ______________________________

   ____ No

2. "Has anything *very bad* happened during the past month—something that worried you a great deal or made you feel a lot worse?"
___Yes (Specify): ________________________________

________________________________

___No

3-8. SIGNIFICANT STRESSFUL OR THREATENING EPISODES OR DEVELOPMENTS IN PATIENT'S LIFE SITUATION DURING PRECEDING MONTH

(These six questions are a further exploration of item 2. Re-enter in these items, if and where appropriate, any "Yes" answer already obtained for item 2. When interrogating, repeat "past month" phrase as needed to maintain time span.)

"Has anything happened . . . (insert wordings below) to cause you a lot of worry or stress and strain?"

3. Interpersonal
"... in your relations with other people at home or outside your home . . ."
(Examples: Hostile clashes, alienation, "in-law trouble," others' illness or death, trouble with children, loneliness.)
(Exceptions: record marital or sexual problems in item 4; record job problems in item 6.)
___Yes ___No

4. Marital and sexual
". . .in your relations with your husband (wife) . . ."
—or (if unmarried)—
". . .in your relations with people of the opposite sex. . ."
(Examples: hostile clashes, alienation, mate's drinking or infidelity, trouble in sex relations, death or illness of mate, divorce or separation, pregnancy of wife or girl friend if cause for undue concern.)
___Yes ___No

5. Economic and domestic
". . .regarding money problems or keeping house or managing things at home . . ."
(Examples: financial setback, excessive debt, spouse's irresponsibility, increase of home duties, unfavorable change of residence.)
(Exception: record job problems in item 6.)
___Yes ___No

6. Occupational
   "...on your job or with people you work with ..."
   –or (if unemployed)–
   "...in connection with trying to get a job, or being out of work ..."
   (Examples: loss of job, frustration in seeking work, demotion, intolerable responsibilities in job, interpersonal trouble at work.)
   ____Yes ____No

7. Social and recreational
   "...in your life in the community, or in church, or in your free-time activities ..."
   (Examples: loss of status in community or civic circles, public embarrassment, trouble with church or religion, frustration in pursuit of hobby, trouble with law.)
   ____Yes ____No

8. Physical health
   "...in connection with your health or physical condition ..."
   (Examples: illness, operation, injury, marked weight loss; pregnancy, if female and with physical or emotional complications; side-effects from medication.)
   (Exception: do not record subjective concern over health without some evidence that concern is realistic.)
   ____Yes ____No

Appendix K

# *Operational Conditions Not Subject to Complete Control in Data Collection

Psychology has ample evidence that situational factors within the observer-subject relationship, functioning as extraneous independent or intervening variables, can systematically affect measurements. We present below some nonconclusive descriptive data on several such variables in the present study. While the study was not designed to assay the effects of such situational factors, the data will supplement our description of research procedures and our discussion of psychometric and logistical issues. The same information may also be useful to others in planning similar surveys or in testing hypotheses concerning situational effects on measurement.

## TIME ELAPSING BETWEEN SUCCESSIVE MONTHLY TESTS

Table K-1 is based on a random sample of tests paired for adjacency. The sample was apportioned approximately equally among the eleven possible adjacencies, i.e., Months 1 and 2, 2 and 3, and so on. Relapse tests were excluded because their timing was not subject to the monthly schedule.

The median number of days between tests is 29.5. In 76 per cent of the pairs, the second test was not more than five days early or late, in terms of the optimum 30-day interval.

# APPENDIX K

*Table K-1. Time Elapsing between Successive Monthly Tests (N = 50 Pairs)*

| Days between Tests | Pairs *N* | Pairs Per Cent |
|---|---|---|
| 40 | 2 | 4 |
| 35-39 | 6 | 12 |
| 30-34 | 17 | 34 |
| 25-29 | 21 | 42 |
| 20-24 | 4 | 8 |
| Total | 50 | 100 |

## PLACE OF TESTING

Most participants chose either to come to our offices for testing or to have the Examiner visit them at home. At Month 1, the only time when all cases could be compared across the board, the distribution of place of testing was essentially the same for each of the three subdivisions of the total sample, and most tests were given in research office quarters (see Table K-2). After Month 1,

*Table K-2. Place of Testing for Month 1: All Cases*

| Place | Complete | | Semicomplete | | Incomplete | | Total | |
|---|---|---|---|---|---|---|---|---|
| | *N* | Per Cent | *N* | Per Cent | *N* | Per Cent | *N* | Per Cent |
| Research office | 28 | 31 | 6 | 21 | 6 | 32 | 40 | 28.8 |
| Research office via clinic[a] | 26 | 29 | 8 | 28 | 4 | 21 | 38 | 27.3 |
| Home of patient and/or informant | 26 | 29 | 11 | 38 | 7 | 37 | 44 | 31.7 |
| All other[b] | 11 | 12 | 4 | 14 | 2 | 11 | 17 | 12.2 |
| Total | 91 | ÷100 | 29 | ÷100 | 19 | ÷100 | 139 | 100.0 |

$\chi^2 = 2.06, p < .95$

[a]Test appointment prearranged on same day as outpatient clinic appointment, in same building, usually immediately following clinic visit. On rare occasions in both of the "Research office" categories, tests had to be given in borrowed quarters near by, in order to solve temporary space problems.

[b]Limited with one exception to occasions where patient and informant were tested at different places (exception: a semicomplete case where Test 1 was a relapse test, administered to both parties in patient's inpatient ward setting). For the three patient groups combined, the remaining "all other" place frequencies were as follows, patient frequency shown first: Research office–5, 4; research office via clinic–4, 0; home of patient and/or informant–1, 12; inpatient setting–3, 0; elsewhere–3, 0; total–16, 16.

when we no longer preferred our own offices as the place for the evaluations, the participants favored their own homes (Tables K-3

*Table K-3. Place of Testing for Month 6: Complete Cases*[a]

| Place | $N$ | Per Cent |
|---|---|---|
| Research office | 12 | 16 |
| Research office via clinic | 12 | 16 |
| Home of patient and/or informant | 40 | 53 |
| All other | 12[b] | 16 |
| Total | 76 | ∻100 |

[a]Fifteen complete cases, not shown, missed Test 6–in most instances because of rehospitalization. Semicomplete and incomplete cases are not tabulated because only four of the former and five of the latter took Test 6.

[b]Ten cases, patient and informant tested at different places; two cases, "elsewhere."

and K-4). At Month 12 (Table K-4), there was again no appreciable difference, in place tested, between the "complete" group and the remainder of those who took this test. It was our impression, not checked statistically, that most participants settled on a preferred appointment location at Month 1 or 2 and thereafter rarely changed to another place.

*Table K-4. Place of Testing for Month 12: Complete and Semicomplete Cases*

| Place | Complete | | Semicomplete | | Total | |
|---|---|---|---|---|---|---|
| | $N$ | Per Cent | $N$ | Per Cent | $N$ | Per Cent |
| Research office (only, or via clinic) | 16 | 22 | 5 | 19 | 21 | 21 |
| Home of patient and/or informant | 43 | 60 | 17 | 65 | 60 | 61 |
| All other[a] | 13 | 18 | 4 | 15 | 17 | 17 |
| Total | 72[b] | 100 | 26[b] | ∻100 | 98 | ∻100 |

$\chi^2 = 0.26, p < .90$

[a]Fourteen cases, patient and informant tested at different places; three cases, all in complete group, elsewhere.

[b]Nineteen complete and three semicomplete cases, not shown, missed Test 12 because of rehospitalization.

## APPENDIX K

# EXAMINERS

The task of conducting our tests and interviews was apportioned quite unequally among eight examiners, identified in Table K-5 by the letters A through H. All of these persons were full-time

*Table K-5. Total Patient-plus-Informant Tests Administered by Each Examiner: Entire Project*

| Examiner | | Tests administered | | |
|---|---|---|---|---|
| | | | Per Cent | |
| Code-Name | Sex | *N* | Each | Cumulative |
| A | Male | 276 | 26.0 | 26.0 |
| B | Female | 267 | 25.1 | 51.1 |
| C | Male | 180 | 16.9 | 68.0 |
| D | Male | 157 | 14.8 | 82.8 |
| E | Male | 136 | 12.8 | 95.6 |
| F | Female | 16 | 1.5 | 97.1 |
| G | Male | 15 | 1.4 | 98.5 |
| H | Female | 15 | 1.4 | ≑100.0 |
| Total | | 1062 | ≑100.0 | – |

*Note*: Based on records for informant tests. Count based on patient tests (not shown) differs negligibly from above, because of occasional examiner changes within single sessions and also because of slight variations in tests missed by patients cf. informants. The above count, as well as the alternate count of patient tests, is actually slightly in excess of the actual total number of "patient-plus-informant tests," because it includes a very few instances where a test was missed by one respondent but taken by the other.

research personnel. Examiners A through E, who carried the bulk of the caseload, were young project-staff employees, all in their twenties. Examiners F, G, and H served only as emergency substitutes. Of all eight examiners, only one, G, worked on the project staff throughout the entire 29-month period of data collection.

As Table K-5 indicates, tests given by males outnumbered those of females by more than two to one. The three most productive examiners—A, B, and C—accounted for a little over two-thirds of the total test data.

A second way of looking at the examiner as an uncontrolled variable is to ask: To what extent did our subjects undergo changes of examiner from month to month? For the average subject, we used from two to three different persons to complete the year-long examiner mission (Table K-6). The psychometric ideal of the constant examiner was rarely attained—in 13.7 per cent of our total sample, but in only 3 per cent of the oft-tested "complete" group. Not surprisingly, changes of examiner became more frequent as more data per case were collected; the "complete" group had the highest rate of change while the incompletes had the lowest.

*Table K-6. Number of Different Examiners Used per Case to Administer All Obtained Tests*

| No. of Examiners | Complete | | Semicomplete | | Incomplete | | Total | |
|---|---|---|---|---|---|---|---|---|
| | *N* | Per Cent | *N* | Per Cent | *N* | Per Cent | *N* | Per Cent |
| One | 3 | 3 | 4 | 14 | 12 | 63 | 19 | 13.7 |
| Two | 25 | 27 | 16 | 55 | 3 | 16 | 44 | 31.7 |
| Three | 38 | 42 | 9 | 31 | 3 | 16 | 50 | 36.0 |
| Four | 18 | 20 | 0 | 0 | 1 | 5 | 19 | 13.7 |
| Five | 7 | 8 | 0 | 0 | 0 | 0 | 7 | 5.0 |
| Total | 91 | 100 | 29 | 100 | 19 | 100 | 139 | ≑100.0 |
| Median | 3.0 | | 2.2 | | 1.3 | | 2.6 | |

*Note*: Based on records for informant tests. Count for patient tests differs negligibly from above.

## INFORMANTS

Informants, though of course more diverse than examiners, were considerably less subject to change of identity during the follow-up year (Table K-7). For nearly three-fourths of all cases,

*Table K-7. Number of Different Informants Used per Patient to Complete All Obtained Informant Tests*

| No. of Informants | Complete | | Semicomplete | | Incomplete | | Total | |
|---|---|---|---|---|---|---|---|---|
| | *N* | Per Cent | *N* | Per Cent | *N* | Per Cent | *N* | Per Cent |
| One | 68 | 75 | 19 | 66 | 16 | 84 | 103 | 74.1 |
| Two | 18 | 20 | 9 | 31 | 3 | 16 | 30 | 21.6 |
| Three | 4 | 4 | 1 | 3 | 0 | 0 | 5 | 3.6 |
| Four | 1 | 1 | 0 | 0 | 0 | 0 | 1 | 0.7 |
| Total | 91 | 100 | 29 | 100 | 19 | 100 | 139 | 100.0 |
| Median | 1.2 | | 1.3 | | 1.1 | | 1.2 | |

one informant accounted for all evaluations. The use of more than two informants for any patient was quite rare. Moreover, the informant's identity—unlike the examiner's—showed no marked or consistent tendency to change as the amount of obtained data increased. Most of the new replacements appropriately reflected major changes in the patient's social environment, as in the case presented in Appendix C where the patient moved out of optimum contact with her original informant.

In view of the comparative stability of the informant's identity, Month-1 data can be taken as reasonably representative of the study as a whole. Table K-8 shows that at this stage half of the

*Table K-8. Relation of Month-1 Informant to Patient*

| Relation | Complete | | Semicomplete | | Incomplete | | Total | |
|---|---|---|---|---|---|---|---|---|
| | *N* | Per Cent | *N* | Per Cent | *N* | Per Cent | *N* | Per Cent |
| Spouse | 46 | 51 | 13 | 45 | 10 | 53 | 69 | 49.6 |
| Mother | 12 | 13 | 7 | 24 | 2 | 11 | 21 | 15.1 |
| All other[a] | 33 | 37 | 9 | 31 | 7 | 37 | 49 | 35.3 |
| Total | 91 | ∸100 | 29 | 100 | 19 | ∸100 | 139 | ∸100.0 |

$\chi^2 = 1.98, p < .75$

[a]Frequencies for all three groups combined: father, 7; son, 3; daughter, 9; brother, 4; sister, 10; other male, 4; other female, 12.

informants were spouses of the patients and all but 11.5 per cent (4 "other male" plus 12 "other female") were close relatives. The complete, semicomplete, and incomplete groups did not differ significantly on informant-patient relationship. The sex distribution of the 139 Month-1 informants, not shown in the table, was 70 males (50.4 per cent) and 69 females (49.6 per cent).

Four out of five informants at Month 1 lived under the same roof with the patient—a condition self-evidently favorable to valid reporting (Table K-9). On this variable there were again no appreciable inter-group differences.

By a clear majority, the patient's closest living relative was likely to be the person who served initially as informant (Table K-10). When the closest living relative was the husband or wife, the tendency for that person to become the informant was about

*Table K-9. Proximity of Month-1 Informant to Patient*

| Proximity | Complete | | Semicomplete | | Incomplete | | Total | |
|---|---|---|---|---|---|---|---|---|
| | N | Per Cent | N | Per Cent | N | Per Cent | N | Per Cent |
| Shared home with patient | 72 | 79 | 26 | 90 | 15 | 79 | 113 | 81 |
| Did not share home | 19 | 21 | 3 | 10 | 4 | 21 | 26 | 19 |
| Total | 91 | 100 | 29 | 100 | 19 | 100 | 139 | 100 |

$\chi^2 = 1.68, p < .50$

*Table K-10. Prevalence of Closest Living Relatives among Informants at Month 1 (Participants, N = 139)*

| Informant | Patient's Closest Living Relative | | | | | | | |
|---|---|---|---|---|---|---|---|---|
| | Spouse | | Parent | | All other | | Total | |
| | N | Per Cent | N | Per Cent | N | Per Cent | N | Per Cent |
| Same person as closest living relative | 69 | 67 | 19 | 66 | 3 | 43 | 91 | 65.5 |
| Other than closest living relative | 34 | 33 | 10 | 34 | 4 | 57 | 48 | 34.5 |
| Total | 103 | 100 | 29 | 100 | 7 | 100 | 139 | 100.0 |

$\chi^2 = 0.41, p < .70$
"Parent" and "all other" columns pooled

the same as when anyone other than a spouse was the closest relative. The fact that many of the closest relatives were working and could not spare time for the study may have been a major reason for the presence of other persons as informants in 34.5 per cent of the cases.

Appendix L

# Distribution of Participants by Specific Diagnosis

This table supplements the diagnostic data in Table II-2 by indicating (1) specific diagnoses rather than gross categories, and (2) distributions for the complete, semicomplete, and incomplete subgroups, in addition to the total participant distribution.

*Table L-1. Final Pre-study Hospital Diagnosis: All Cases*

| Diagnosis | Complete | | Semicomplete | | Incomplete | | Total | |
|---|---|---|---|---|---|---|---|---|
| | *N* | Per Cent | *N* | Per Cent | *N* | Per Cent | *N* | Per Cent |
| Psychotic disorders | | | | | | | | |
| Involutional psychotic reaction | 8 | 9 | 3 | 10 | 3 | 16 | 14 | 10.1 |
| Affective reactions | | | | | | | | |
| Manic depressive reaction, manic type | | | 1 | 3 | 1 | 5 | 2 | 1.4 |
| Manic depressive reaction, depressive type | 4 | 4 | 1 | 3 | | | 5 | 3.6 |
| Manic depressive reaction, other | 1 | 1 | | | | | 1 | 0.7 |
| Psychotic depressive reaction | 4 | 4 | | | 1 | 5 | 5 | 3.6 |
| Schizophrenic reactions | | | | | | | | |
| Schizophrenic reaction, simple type | 1 | 1 | | | | | 1 | 0.7 |
| Schizophrenic reaction, hebephrenic type | 2 | 2 | | | 1 | 5 | 3 | 2.2 |

*(Table L-1, continued)*

| Diagnosis | Complete | | Semicomplete | | Incomplete | | Total | |
|---|---|---|---|---|---|---|---|---|
| | N | Per Cent | N | Per Cent | N | Per Cent | N | Per Cent |
| Schizophrenic reaction, catatonic type | 3 | 3 | | | 1 | 5 | 4 | 2.9 |
| Schizophrenic reaction, paranoid type | 17 | 19 | 6 | 21 | 4 | 21 | 27 | 19.4 |
| Schizophrenic reaction, acute undifferentiated type | 7 | 8 | | | | | 7 | 5.0 |
| Schizophrenic reaction, chronic undifferentiated type | 20 | 22 | 8 | 28 | 3 | 16 | 31 | 22.3 |
| Schizophrenic reaction, schizo-affective type | 2 | 2 | | | 1 | 5 | 3 | 2.2 |
| Paranoid reactions | | | | | | | | |
| Subdivision not specified | 1 | 1 | | | | | 1 | 0.7 |
| Psychoneurotic disorders | | | | | | | | |
| Psychoneurotic reactions | | | | | | | | |
| Anxiety reaction | 1 | 1 | 2 | 7 | | | 3 | 2.2 |
| Conversion reaction | 1 | 1 | 1 | 3 | | | 2 | 1.4 |
| Depressive reaction | 12 | 13 | 5 | 17 | 2 | 11 | 19 | 13.7 |
| Personality disorders | | | | | | | | |
| Personality pattern disturbance | | | | | | | | |
| Inadequate personality | 1 | 1 | | | 1 | 5 | 2 | 1.4 |
| Schizoid personality | 1 | 1 | | | | | 1 | 0.7 |
| Personality trait disturbance | | | | | | | | |
| Emotionally unstable personality | 1 | 1 | | | | | 1 | 0.7 |
| Passive-aggressive personality | 2 | 2 | | | | | 2 | 1.4 |
| Compulsive personality | 1 | 1 | | | | | 1 | 0.7 |
| Sociopathic personality disturbance | | | | | | | | |
| Antisocial reaction | | | 1 | 3 | | | 1 | 0.7 |
| Dyssocial reaction | | | | | 1 | 5 | 1 | 0.7 |
| Transient situational personality disorders | | | | | | | | |
| Transient situational personality disturbance | | | | | | | | |
| Adult situational reaction | | | 1 | 3 | | | 1 | 0.7 |
| Adjustment reaction of late life | 1 | 1 | | | | | 1 | 0.7 |
| Total | 91 | ∸100 | 29 | ∸100 | 19 | ∸100 | 139 | ∸100.0 |

Appendix M

# Interrelationships among the 26 Adjustment Variables

Table M-1 presents the master correlation matrix for all adjustment variables at Month 1, together with a Month-12 replication. At Month 12, *N* dwindles to 94 mainly because of missed tests; in addition, we have excluded four cases whose 12th test was a relapse test, so as to cover in-community adjustment more representatively.

To aid in inspecting and evaluating these results, we have sorted the correlations into eight conceptually discrete categories. Table M-2 defines the categories and extracts some of the trends to be noted in Table M-1.

*Table M-1. Adjustment Variables: Significant Intercorrelations at Months 1 and 12*

| Variable | Patient KAS | | | | | | Informant KAS R1 | | | | | | | | | | | | | Informant KAS R2 to 5 | | | | | Stress | |
|---|---|---|---|---|---|---|---|---|---|---|---|---|---|---|---|---|---|---|---|---|---|---|---|---|---|---|
| | *Sym* | *SEA-P* | *LOE-P* | *SSA-P* | *FTA-P* | *SFA-P* | *Bel* | *Exp* | *Neg* | *Hel* | *Sus* | *Anx* | *Wdl* | *Psy* | *Ner* | *Con* | *Biz* | *Hyp* | *Sta* | *SEA-I* | *LOE-I* | *SSA-I* | *FTA-I* | *SFA-I* | *Str-P* | *Str-I* |
| Patient KAS | | | | | | | | | | | | | | | | | | | | | | | | | | |
| *Sym* | | .22 | * | .35 | * | .32 | .18 | * | .17 | .33 | .18 | .34 | * | .29 | .41 | .27 | .19 | .23 | .21 | * | * | * | * | * | .53 | .32 |
| *SEA-P* | .27 | | .70 | .56 | .47 | .17 | .17 | * | .28 | .30 | .18 | * | .37 | .31 | .24 | .21 | * | .23 | .39 | .56 | .38 | .34 | .29 | .25 | * | * |
| *LOE-P* | * | .66 | | * | .46 | * | .22 | * | .29 | .24 | * | * | .36 | .26 | .18 | * | * | .17 | .33 | .47 | .40 | .25 | .28 | * | * | * |
| *SSA-P* | .29 | .57 | * | | * | .19 | * | * | * | .17 | * | * | * | * | .18 | .18 | * | .18 | * | .22 | * | .19 | * | .27 | .23 | * |
| *FTA-P* | .22 | .47 | .40 | * | | * | * | * | .19 | .26 | * | * | .37 | .21 | .17 | .24 | .19 | .18 | .32 | .36 | .26 | .30 | .39 | .22 | * | * |
| *SFA-P* | .40 | * | * | .23 | * | | * | * | * | .17 | .17 | * | * | .18 | * | .28 | * | * | * | * | * | * | .25 | .21 | .27 | * |
| Informant KAS R1 | | | | | | | | | | | | | | | | | | | | | | | | | | |
| *Bel* | * | * | * | * | * | * | | .52 | .61 | .51 | .58 | .54 | * | .67 | .46 | .42 | .50 | .45 | .23 | .31 | .26 | * | * | .20 | .22 | .30 |
| *Exp* | * | * | * | * | * | * | .78 | | .47 | .37 | .49 | .45 | * | .57 | .32 | .26 | .39 | .40 | * | * | * | * | * | * | * | .21 |
| *Neg* | * | * | * | * | * | * | .74 | .81 | | .63 | .61 | .49 | .47 | .80 | .58 | .30 | .45 | .49 | .58 | .47 | .33 | .23 | .33 | .43 | .19 | .23 |
| *Hel* | * | * | * | .22 | * | * | .66 | .75 | .70 | | .58 | .70 | .52 | .76 | .63 | .42 | .60 | .55 | .49 | .55 | .38 | .30 | .41 | .51 | .25 | .35 |
| *Sus* | * | * | * | * | * | * | .74 | .73 | .65 | .69 | | .64 | .22 | .74 | .58 | .46 | .67 | .50 | .25 | .39 | .25 | .17 | .22 | .26 | .27 | .30 |
| *Anx* | * | * | * | .25 | * | * | .68 | .64 | .61 | .76 | .71 | | .22 | .69 | .67 | .48 | .68 | .56 | .29 | .28 | .17 | .18 | .21 | .28 | .18 | .33 |
| *Wdl* | * | .37 | .24 | .31 | * | * | .29 | .36 | .32 | .62 | .42 | .49 | | .43 | .36 | * | .19 | .22 | .39 | .57 | .44 | .34 | .44 | .49 | * | * |
| *Psy* | * | * | * | * | * | * | .75 | .81 | .79 | .80 | .75 | .71 | .56 | | .71 | .41 | .61 | .62 | .46 | .52 | .35 | .29 | .37 | .47 | .30 | .35 |
| *Ner* | * | * | * | * | * | * | .45 | .55 | .50 | .63 | .56 | .68 | .52 | .69 | | .34 | .48 | .65 | .36 | .35 | .24 | * | .29 | .38 | .24 | .40 |
| *Con* | * | * | * | * | * | .20 | .33 | .26 | .23 | .30 | .32 | .30 | .23 | .29 | * | | .55 | .34 | * | .25 | * | .26 | * | .26 | * | .27 |
| *Biz* | * | * | * | .24 | * | * | .78 | .75 | .67 | .78 | .79 | .70 | .47 | .73 | .44 | .42 | | .48 | .27 | .31 | .20 | * | .22 | .25 | .19 | .34 |
| *Hyp* | * | .23 | .23 | * | * | * | .63 | .63 | .64 | .70 | .62 | .59 | .53 | .80 | .54 | .37 | .68 | | .31 | .29 | .17 | .18 | .25 | .33 | .24 | .34 |
| *Sta* | * | * | * | .22 | * | * | .43 | .45 | .67 | .47 | .43 | .44 | .34 | .54 | .34 | * | .46 | .57 | | .48 | .35 | .29 | .30 | .42 | .21 | * |
| Informant KAS R2 … 5 | | | | | | | | | | | | | | | | | | | | | | | | | | |
| *SEA-I* | * | .49 | .30 | .38 | .22 | * | .33 | .33 | .43 | .44 | .39 | .34 | .54 | .53 | .35 | * | .42 | .54 | .60 | | .68 | .53 | .57 | .51 | * | * |
| *LOE-I* | * | .31 | .32 | * | * | * | * | * | * | * | * | * | .20 | * | * | * | * | .29 | .26 | .61 | | * | .36 | .22 | * | * |
| *SSA-I* | .20 | .30 | * | .44 | * | * | .48 | .53 | .47 | .54 | .45 | .43 | .52 | .57 | .42 | * | .51 | .45 | .51 | .65 | * | | .35 | .49 | * | .26 |
| *FTA-I* | * | .33 | * | .28 | .31 | * | * | * | .28 | .30 | .28 | .24 | .45 | .36 | .30 | * | .24 | .37 | .39 | .69 | .47 | .45 | | .48 | * | * |
| *SFA-I* | * | .22 | * | .22 | * | * | .38 | .46 | .48 | .59 | .40 | .48 | .52 | .61 | .53 | * | .44 | .47 | .55 | .55 | * | .66 | .44 | | * | * |
| Stress | | | | | | | | | | | | | | | | | | | | | | | | | | |
| *Str-P* | .35 | * | * | * | .20 | * | * | * | * | * | * | * | * | * | * | * | * | * | * | * | * | * | * | * | | .55 |
| *Str-I* | .34 | * | * | .24 | * | * | .37 | .29 | .38 | .27 | .32 | .29 | * | .41 | * | * | .28 | .27 | .28 | .21 | * | .29 | * | * | .70 | |

*Note:* Month 1 above diagonal, $N = 139$ participants; Month 12 below diagonal, $N = 94$ participants who took Test 12. Asterisk * indicates correlation omitted because *not* significant at .05 level by two-tailed test. At Month 1 the minimum $r$ values for significance are $\pm.17$ ($p = .05$) and $\pm.22$ ($p = .01$); corresponding values at Month 12 are $\pm.20$ and $\pm.25$. The fact that all the significant $r$s are positive means that favorable scores on each $X$ variable are consistently associated with favorable $Y$ scores and conversely; in the original results, minus signs (omitted here) occurred wherever the $X$ and $Y$ scales differed as to favorable-unfavorable direction.

*Table M-2. Adjustment Variables at Months 1 and 12: Interpretive Summary of Intercorrelations in Table M-1*

| *X* Variables•*Y* Variables | Import of *r* Results | Total No. of *r*s Each Month | Per Cent of *r*s Significant | | Largest Single *r* | |
|---|---|---|---|---|---|---|
| | | | Month 1 | Month 12 | Month 1 | Month 12 |
| 1. Patient KAS and Patient stress•*matching* informant KAS and informant stress[a] | Interrespondent agreement | 6 | 100 | 83 | .56 | .70 |
| 2a. Patient KAS•Patient KAS | Interrelations among adjustment | 15 | 60 | 60 | .70 | .66 |
| 2b. Informant KAS•Informant KAS | variables (within same respondent) | 153 | 88.9 | 86.9 | .80 | .81 |
| 3. Patient KAS•*nonmatching* informant KAS[b] | Interrelations among adjustment variables (criss-crossing respondents) | 103 | 58.3 | 19.4 | .47 | .38 |
| 4a. Patient stress•Patient KAS | Relation of stress to adjustment | 6 | 50 | 33 | .53 | .35 |
| 4b. Informant stress•Informant KAS | (within same respondent) | 18 | 67 | 67 | .40 | .41 |
| 5a. Patient stress•Informant KAS | Relation of stress to adjustment | 18 | 56 | 0 | .30 | .17 |
| 5b. Informant stress•Patient KAS | (criss-crossing respondents) | 6 | 17 | 33 | .32 | .34 |
| Total | | 325 | 72.9 | 56.3 | | |

[a]Scales *SEA, LOE, SSA, FTA, SFA,* and *Str* were administered both to patients and informants in virtually identical forms. These are the correlations for the matching forms, e.g. *SEA-P•SEA-I.*

[b]Every patient KAS measure intercorrelated with every informant KAS measure, except for the matching forms covered in section 1 of the table.

Appendix N

# *Detailed Statistics Pertaining to Sampling Bias

The main lineaments of our findings on sampling bias are noted and discussed at the end of Chapter II. To provide the essential documentation, we present below the complete results of our sampling bias analyses.

---

## PARTICIPANTS COMPARED WITH REFERENCE POPULATION

The Maryland Psychiatric Case Register issues frequent reports, some regular and some special, on the operations of the state's treatment system. In Table N-1, compiled in part from one of the Register's special reports, most of the participants are compared with a larger group of Spring Grove ex-patients which must have closely resembled our true reference population. Comparisons were possible on 5 of our 12 Background variables. Additionally, sex differences on each variable were tested within each group and significance levels are shown. In general, the two groups were quite similar as to direction of sex differences (not tabulated)—strikingly so on Age and Years of education. The greatest discrepancy was observed on No. of hospitalizations prior to last: male percentages for Case Register patients and participants respectively were:

*Table N-1. Participants Compared with Larger Spring Grove Cohort Followed by Maryland Psychiatric Case Register*

| Variable | Case Register[a] | | | Participants[b] | | |
|---|---|---|---|---|---|---|
| | *N* | Per Cent | Sex Differences:[c] *p* | *N* | Per Cent | Sex Differences:[c] *p* |
| Age | | | | | | |
| 25 to 34 | 311 | 34.0 | .05 | 36 | 34.0 | .01 |
| 35 to 44 | 358 | 39.1 | | 32 | 30.2 | |
| 45 to 54 | 246 | 26.9 | | 38 | 35.8 | |
| Total | 915 | 100.0 | | 106 | 100.0 | |
| Marital status | | | | | | |
| Single | 166 | 19.0 | .001 | 16 | 15.1 | .001 |
| Married | 488 | 55.8 | | 75 | 70.8 | |
| All other | 221 | 25.3 | | 15 | 14.2 | |
| Total | 875 | ≑100.0 | | 106 | ≑100.0 | |
| Years of education | | | | | | |
| Less than 9 | 293 | 32.8 | .001 | 30 | 28.3 | .01 |
| 9 to 12 | 477 | 53.4 | | 64 | 60.4 | |
| 13 or more | 123 | 13.8 | | 12 | 11.3 | |
| Total | 893 | 100.0 | | 106 | 100.0 | |
| No. of hospitalizations prior to last | | | | | | |
| None | 447 | 48.9 | .10 | 31 | 29.2 | .70 |
| One | 278 | 30.4 | | 26 | 24.8 | |
| Two or more | 190 | 20.8 | | 49 | 46.2 | |
| Total | 915 | ≑100.0 | | 106 | ≑100.0 | |

*(Table N-1, continued)*

| Variable | Case Register[a] | | | Participants[b] | | |
|---|---|---|---|---|---|---|
| | $N$ | Per Cent | Sex Differences:[c] $p$ | $N$ | Per Cent | Sex Differences:[c] $p$ |
| Diagnosis | | | | | | |
| Psychotic | 615 | 67.2 | .99 | 82 | 77.4 | .80 |
| Nonpsychotic | 300 | 32.8 | | 24 | 22.6 | |
| Total | 915 | 100.0 | | 106 | 100.0 | |

[a]Data are for Spring Grove, extracted from a cohort follow-up study which overlapped our own in posthospital calendar time (U.S. Department of Health, Education and Welfare, and Maryland Department of Mental Hygiene, 1966); Case Register selection criteria were closely similar to our own, and *all* eligible patients were studied.

[b]Total sample truncated here by age in order to match Case Register sample's age range of 25 to 54.

[c]Based on male-female frequencies not shown.

None, 47.6 per cent *vs.* 30; one, 28.0 per cent vs. 18; two or more, 24.4 per cent *vs.* 52. (See Table II-4 for sex-difference findings on all 139 participants.)

Among the 139 participants, females outnumbered males more than two to one. The reference population, however, appears to have contained a similar imbalance, perhaps favoring females slightly less heavily. Controlling for race and diagnosis as in the study sample, we find that 61.6 per cent of all 778 such patients on leave from Spring Grove as of July 1, 1963, were females (U. S. Department of Health, Education, and Welfare, and Maryland State Department of Mental Hygiene, 1964). (In Maryland *admission* rates, on the other hand, men exceed women: Five out of every six alcoholics are male, and alcoholism has the highest admission rate of all the major diagnostic categories (Gorwitz, Bahn, Klee, and Solomon, 1966, p. 1103).)

## PARTICIPANTS COMPARED WITH NONPARTICIPANTS

The 12 background variables comprised the only data originally available for comparing participants with nonparticipants. Differences on age and education were tested by $t$; chi square was used for the other 10 variables. Participants tended more often to be married and to have more children; when leaving Spring Grove, they were much more often placed on convalescent leave (as opposed to being discharged outright) than were nonparticipants (Table N-2). Among the nine remaining background variables, the most nearly significant difference was on education, where participants were slightly higher ($p < .30$). All other $p$ values were greater than .40 and most were greater than .70.

## COMPLETES COMPARED WITH NONPARTICIPANTS: BACKGROUND AND RELATED VARIABLES

Of prime importance are similarities and/or differences between the 91 completes and 79 nonparticipants, inasmuch as the former are the source of the study's most intensive substantive findings. On background variables, comparison results were expectedly quite similar to those in Table N-2; $p$ values for the three most

*Table N-2. Background Variables Showing Greatest Differences between Participants (N = 139) and Nonparticipants (N = 79)*

| Item | Participants | | Nonparticipants | |
|---|---|---|---|---|
| | *N* | Per Cent | *N* | Per Cent |
| Marital status ($p < .20$): | | | | |
| Single | 24 | 17.3 | 21 | 27 |
| Married | 87 | 62.6 | 35 | 44 |
| Widowed | 5 | 3.6 | 4 | 5 |
| Separated | 17 | 12.2 | 14 | 18 |
| Divorced | 6 | 4.3 | 5 | 6 |
| Number of children ($p < .10$): | | | | |
| None | 36 | 25.9 | 31 | 39 |
| One | 23 | 16.5 | 16 | 20 |
| Two | 36 | 25.9 | 10 | 13 |
| Three | 25 | 18.0 | 10 | 13 |
| Four or more | 19 | 13.7 | 12 | 15 |
| Type of release ($p < .001$): | | | | |
| Convalescent leave | 115 | 82.7 | 47 | 59 |
| Discharge, doctor's consent | 24 | 17.3 | 32 | 41 |

significant differences were identical except for marital status, which here was at the .10 level.[1]

Several steps, described in this and the following section, were taken in order to obtain the most definitive possible comparisons of completes with nonparticipants. All of these steps involved the collection of additional data beyond that available in the study proper. The first operation was to compile three additional clinical background variables from hospital records. Results are presented in Table N-3; despite their lack of significance, they serve to augment descriptive information on the "complete" group. To test more precisely for the difference on prognosis, for which chi square had indicated $p < .10$, we converted the ratings to a four-point scale and tested mean differences by $t$. The result was 1.29, $p < .30$.

[1]Completes and nonparticipants differed negligibly as to diagnosis ($p < .70$). Two additional checks on diagnosis were made by comparing both groups with an approximated reference population of 1,495 ex-patients based on Maryland Psychiatric Case Register statistics (U.S. Department of Health, Education, and Welfare, and Maryland State Department of Mental Hygiene, 1964). The completes were found to be slightly overweighted with nonschizophrenic psychotics ($p < .20$). Nonparticipants were diagnostically quite similar to the reference population ($p < .90$).

*Table N-3. Type of Admission, Prognosis, and Rated Impairment: Complete Group (N = 91) Compared with Nonparticipants (N = 79)*

| Item | Complete | | Nonparticipant | |
|---|---|---|---|---|
| | *N* | Per Cent | *N* | Per Cent |
| Type of admission ($p < .90$): | | | | |
| Civil: two medical certificates | 39 | 43 | 38 | 49 |
| Return from convalescent leave | 24 | 26 | 21 | 27 |
| Voluntary | 22 | 24 | 15 | 19 |
| Return from elopement | 6 | 7 | 4 | 5 |
| Total | 91 | 100 | 78 | 100 |
| Prognosis when released ($p < .10$): | | | | |
| Poor | 2 | 4 | 2 | 4 |
| Guarded | 27 | 47 | 30 | 59 |
| Fair | 14 | 25 | 15 | 29 |
| Good | 14 | 25 | 4 | 8 |
| Total | 57 | ∻100 | 51 | 100 |
| Rated impairment when released ($p < .20$): | | | | |
| Severe | 8 | 15 | 15 | 31 |
| Moderate | 16 | 30 | 11 | 22 |
| Mild | 21 | 39 | 13 | 27 |
| None | 9 | 17 | 10 | 20 |
| Total | 54 | ∻100 | 49 | 100 |

*Note*: All $p$ values based on $\chi^2$; in testing Prognosis, "poor" and "guarded" frequencies were pooled. Shortages in five of the six total *N*s are due to information not being in charts at time of data collection, plus temporary unavailability of one chart.

Because data collection required travel and personal contact, we suspected that those patients living farthest from Spring Grove may have tended more often to become nonparticipants. Accordingly, we compared the two groups as to air-miles distance between hospital and home. (Because of the laboriousness of mapping and measuring for each case, we limited this comparison to second-wave cases: $N = 43$ completes, 34 nonparticipants.) The average distance for completes was 13.2 miles, S.D. 8.6, range 1.5 to 36.0; nonparticipants averaged 15.3 miles, S.D. 10.9, range 2.2 to 48.0. The difference, though in the expected direction, was not significant ($t = 0.88, p < .40$).

Using the same second-wave cases, and the same data on location of home, we also tested a rough-hewn ecological hypothesis: that the *direction* of the home location in reference to Spring Grove may have differentially affected study participation.

Dividing the entire patient residential territory into four compass quadrants, we found that 67 per cent of the completes and 56 per cent of the nonparticipants came from the northeastern sector (predominantly urban Baltimore) and none from the southwestern sector, essentially because of catchment area locations. The ecological hypothesis was not supported: $p < .70$.

Another clue toward possible sampling bias was sought in the monthly attrition rate. Did the 91 completes and 79 nonparticipants differ in pace of accession to project rosters? Not significantly so ($p < .25$).

## COMPLETES COMPARED WITH NONPARTICIPANTS: THE NONPARTICIPANT STUDY

Many vital questions about the nonparticipants remained unanswered even after we had considered all of the results hereto reported. In view of the project's high attrition rate, it was clear that the usefulness of its findings would depend substantially on how much we could learn about its "dropouts." Most pressing was the need for whatever information could be garnered concerning their posthospital year. The steps which we took toward meeting this need constituted a special sub-project, dubbed the "Nonparticipant Study."

### *Design and Procedure*

In the Nonparticipant Study we undertook to contact as many of this group as possible after their posthospital year had ended, and to conduct a single carefully designed fact-gathering interview covering retrospectively the entire 12-month period. We relinquished at the outset any intention to measure directly the nonparticipants' posthospital *adjustment*; while many studies have accomplished this with a similar design, we felt that in our case even the best such data attainable would still fail to meet the prime requirement of comparability with the monthly KAS and Stress Index data which the completes had provided us. (For circumstantial and practical reasons a single Month-12 evaluation was out of the question.) The limitation did not apply, however, to most of our matter-of-fact life-situation items, and certainly not to rehospitalization experience.

With this in mind, we carefully constructed a "condensed interview" schedule in such a manner that (1) the entire posthospital year was covered, instead of a single monthly segment as in the main study; (2) major emphasis was on life situation; and (3) yearly coverage was accomplished in such a way that, by condensing analogous monthly longitudinal data on the completes, we could make the two sets of data isomorphic and hence statistically comparable. Detailed features of the condensed interview format and the condensation of completes' data are implicit below in presentations of results.

The standard procedure for recruiting and data collection fell into three phases. (1) The current home address was obtained from the Spring Grove files. (2) With no mention of our previous research overtures, a letter was sent to the patient, saying that the hospital was interested in learning how people got along after leaving it, and that one of its interviewers would be likely to call on him soon within a specified period of three consecutive days. The patient was given the option of telephoning us, collect if necessary, to set a certain hour for the visit and/or to stipulate any meeting place other than his home if he so desired. (3) If there were no complications, the interviewer visited the patient as planned and conducted the condensed interview.

Complications did of course often develop. As expected, nonparticipants were comparatively refractory to the establishment of effective contact–not only pre-selectedly but also because of the longer interval between hospital release and research recruitment. As indicated in Chapter II (Table II-13), face-to-face refusals of the interview were quite rare. More often a patient, failing to respond to our letter, was found to have moved to a new residence, which we made every effort to discover–either with or without benefit of a forwarding address.

Interviewing began in September, 1965, and was completed in January, 1966. Of the total of 79 nonparticipants, we were able to find, persuade, and interview 50.[2] These 50 constituted the sub-

[2]In four instances it was both necessary and practicable to obtain the interview by telephone. In eight other cases, all female, adequate coverage was attainable only by interviewing informants in lieu of patients: five husbands, a mother, a stepmother, and a sister.

group to be called "nonparticipant-seen"; the remaining 29 are designated "nonparticipant-unseen." Most advantageously, the male staff member who conducted nearly all of the condensed interviews had previously served as the busiest of all examiners in the main study. In canvassing nonparticipants, we found that some had been rehospitalized at Spring Grove or elsewhere, and from these patients we were usually able to obtain the interview in their inpatient setting.

*Problems of Veridicality*

We observed a number of safeguards to ensure optimum accuracy of the interview reports, especially regarding the error-prone items covering outpatient and inpatient treatment received during the posthospital year. Individual case records and outpatient appointment rosters were consulted by permission, both at Spring Grove and at other institutions, whenever the interview data were incomplete or questionable. Letters, telephone calls, and personal visits to hospitals and clinics by the interviewer or assistants were freely employed as needed.

The Maryland Psychiatric Case Register was superlatively useful as a further resource for checking interview reports on treatment. The Register had recently begun to maintain computerized case records, individually identifiable and dated, of treatment received in almost all facilities throughout the state excepting clinicians in private practice. By using its printouts on our nonparticipant cases, we had at our disposal official treatment records on all 50 of those who were interviewed, plus 3 who were not.[3]

Possible inaccuracies of respondent memory are crucial to the issue of veridicality. In the main study the maximum time span covered retrospectively in any session was about one month; in the Nonparticipant Study it was more than a year. Ideally, each condensed interview would have been conducted very soon after the end of the posthospital study year. That circumstances decreed otherwise served to aggravate the memory problem. The nonpar-

[3]Thus for some of the treatment data (inpatient and outpatient facilities, but not drug treatment) our total *N* was augmented from 50 to 53. Case Register treatment data were unavailable on the remaining 26 nonparticipants because of posting lag during the early development phase of the Register's record-keeping program.

ticipant study was not even conceived until rather late in our main project; thereafter, not only did it have to be planned and launched, but the 79 subjects had to be contacted anew and searched out when hard to find; following this, interviews had to be "sold," scheduled, and conducted. Time lag mounted beyond the one-year minimum throughout all of these proceedings. Consequently, 16 of the 50 condensed interviews (32 per cent) were completed within three to seven months after the end of the post-hospital year; 15 (30 per cent) within 8 to 17 months; and 19 (38 per cent) within 18 to 22 months. The median time lag from end of year to interview was 14.8 months. Nevertheless, the one meticulous interviewer who saw nearly all of the respondents felt distinctly that their retrospective reports were not appreciably hampered by time lag and memory difficulty. In conducting the interview he was often able to orient and cue the respondent by referring to treatment-history information, etc., which we had compiled beforehand from Spring Grove records and sometimes from additional sources. Moreover, he found respondent accuracy to have been remarkably good when cross-checking from interview reports of treatment to Case Register printouts. Pursuing this question further, we tested some of our data internally for time-lag effects; results are noted at the end of this section.

*Course of Adjustment: Rehospitalization*

In the absence of any KAS scores on nonparticipants, the only intimation of their course of adjustment is to be found in rehospitalization rates (Table N-4). Differences here were neither significant nor consistent: there was no linear trend associated with amount of research participation. With the two nonparticipant subgroups pooled, the complete-*vs.*-nonparticipant difference was again not nearly significant ($p < .50$). Considering only the seen and unseen nonparticipants, one does see in Table N-4 a consistent difference, with the unseens having fewer rehospitalizations; it does not quite reach significance, however ($p < .10$).[4]

[4]On number of rehospitalizations there was little difference also between the 79 nonparticipants and the total study sample of 139 participants: $p < .50$.

*Table N-4. Number of Rehospitalizations in Complete, Nonparticipant-Seen, and Nonparticipant-Unseen Groups*

| No. of Rehospitalizations | Complete | | Nonparticipant | | | |
|---|---|---|---|---|---|---|
| | | | Seen | | Unseen | |
| | *N* | Per Cent | *N* | Per Cent | *N* | Per Cent |
| None | 51 | 56 | 27 | 54 | 22 | 76 |
| One | 33 | 36 | 15 | 30 | 6 | 21 |
| Two to five[a] | 7 | 8 | 8 | 16 | 1 | 3 |
| Total | 91 | 100 | 50 | 100 | 29 | 100 |

$\chi^2 = 7.18, p < .30$

[a]Maximum number of rehospitalizations was two, except for one "Complete" male with three rehospitalizations and one nonparticipant-seen female with five.

We also compared all completes with all nonparticipants as to total number of days rehospitalized. None of the several results approached significance: *p* values varied from .70 to .90, depending on whether *t* or chi square was used and whether all patients or only relapsers were considered.

It is possible that the frequency counts for rehospitalizations in the nonparticipant-unseen group are slightly less than the true values. Except for the three cases reported to us by the Maryland Psychiatric Case Register, our only coverage for rehospitalization in this group was to check admission records at Spring Grove and the other three major state mental hospitals: Crownsville, Springfield, and Eastern Shore.

Beginning here, data from the condensed interview are subject to several fluctuations in *N*. To avoid reportorial tedium, let us state generally the conditions of fluctuation as against our standard *N* of 50 nonparticipants-seen. (1) Months 1 and 12 were the two anchor points for organizing the data. Month-12 data are limited to patients who were *not* at that time on rehospitalized inpatient status (69 completes, 40 nonparticipant-seens). (2) All life situation data are subject to the same attenuations as in the main study (Appendix R). (3) Occasionally data analyses are based on control-variable subgroupings, e.g., by sex and marital status under "work and homemaking." (4) Finally, as previously noted (footnote 3), data on treatment were augmented when possible by inclusion of three nonparticipant-unseen cases covered by the Maryland Psychiatric Case Register.

Statistical comparisons of completes with nonparticipant-seens, starting with the condensed interview data obtained from the latter group, proved to be a painstaking task involving multifarious compilations, editings, rearrangements, final inspections, and analyses of data, and yielding voluminous results. To make the final output more tolerable for readers, we have largely avoided tabular presentations and lengthy qualifications, and have sought maximum condensation below. Thus, terseness of the reporting reflects compression rather than oversight.

*Life Situation: Home and Family*

In this area there were only two significant differences between completes and nonparticipant-seens, out of a total of 14 tested comparisons. Both involved children. To summarize, for the completes there was greater residential movement of blood-related children into ($p < .02$) and out of ($p < .05$) the home—not including children leaving for or returning from college, etc. At Months 1 and 12, however, there was no discrepancy as to number of children, blood-related or otherwise, residing either at home or elsewhere. The remaining nonsignificant differences involved movement of non-blood-related children; type of home (conjugal, etc.) at Months 1 and 12; changes in type of home during the year; and parents living *vs.* deceased.

*Life Situation: Work and Homemaking*

Work was tested in nine analyses and homemaking in three. Possible sampling bias appeared on only 2 of the total 12 comparisons, both pertaining to homemaking. Among the completes, women were shouldering much more responsibility than among nonparticipant-seens at Month 1 ($p < .001$), but at Month 12 the difference had diminished ($p < .20$). "Complete" females also led in frequency of changes in degree of homemaker responsibility throughout the year ($p < .001$).[5]

[5]Veridicality is again problematical for this type of data. Changes during the year may have been more effectively registered by the monthly tests which only the completes had undergone.

Employment outside the home was negative for signs of sampling bias. Differences between the two groups were clearly random for males as well as for nonmarried females. For married females only, completes showed a consistent but nonsignificant ($p < .25$) leaning toward more employment on all three items tested: total months worked during the year, greatest part of any month worked, and highest number of hours on the job in any week.

*Life Situation: Outpatient Treatment*

In this area a noteworthy total of five highly significant differences emerged from the 13 tests made. With one interesting exception, all indicated completes to have been much more densely involved in aftercare treatment than nonparticipant-seens. They more often used two, three, or (rarely) even four separate treatment facilities at some time during the year, while nonparticipant-seens more often used none or only one ($p < .001$). Completes also excelled on three counts of attendance at specific facilities. (1) They used the Spring Grove Outpatient Clinic more often throughout the posthospital year ($p < .005$). (2) At either or both of the anchor months 1 and 12, they were also more often present at the Spring Grove Clinic ($p < .02$). (3) They visited a private nonpsychiatric physician more often during the year ($p < .001$). Paradoxically, however, nonparticipant-seens exceeded completes in physician visits at Month 1 and/or Month 12 ($p < .01$). No appreciable differences were found on use of other treatment facilities: other public clinics, private psychiatrist, visiting public health nurse, "all other."

*Life Situation: Drug Treatment*[6]

Among all of the life situation areas, drug treatment proved most evidently liable to sampling bias. Five out of seven variables tested showed completes to have used drugs decisively more than nonparticipant-seens; all five chi squares reached the .001 level. Ninety-six per cent of all completes took at least some drug during

[6]In order to focus these analyses on actual consumption of drug, we included in the "none" categories not only those patients who had no drug prescribed but also those who, despite having a prescription, reported no medication consumed.

their in-community time, while only 66 per cent of the nonparticipant-seens did so. Completes more often used a drug for all or a large part of Month 1, as well as of their latest in-community month during the year. When they did take medicine, their typical daily consumption during Month 1 (expressed as proportion of prescribed daily dosage) was greater. Likewise greater was their maximum typical daily consumption during any in-community month.

On only two of the drug usage variables, both pertaining to typical daily drug intake, were the significance tests essentially negative. These related to the latest in-community month ($p < .10$, more usage by completes) and to the minimum amount of drug used during any in-community month ($p < .30$).

*Treatment Differences Retested with Type of Release Controlled*

Having now surveyed all of the nonparticipant study findings, we must raise the question: To what extent are some or all of the observed significant differences between completes and nonparticipant-seens merely a function of the antecedent variable, type of release? To explain: Type of release was found to discriminate sharply between completes and nonparticipant-seens ($p < .02$), in the same direction as in Table N-2. It is therefore possible that the comparatively high rate of convalescent leave in the complete group may have automatically predisposed them to the higher rate of aftercare treatment and drug usage reported immediately above. (Spring Grove aftercare policy tends to favor convalescent-leave patients.) We have tested this hypothesis in relation to those outpatient treatment and drug treatment variables where significant and near-significant differences were found. Results indicated in the main that, whenever type of release was demonstrably associated with the aftercare variables, it most often did *not* thereby account for the observed treatment differences between completes and nonparticipant-seens. Hence these differences cannot generally be dismissed as being merely a function of type of release.

Tables N-5, N-6, and N-7 demonstrate for one variable (use of Spring Grove Outpatient Clinic during posthospital year) our three successive steps in testing the type-of-release hypothesis. Step 1 was simply to begin with the significant difference, already re-

*Table N-5. Use of Spring Grove State Hospital Outpatient Clinic during Posthospital Year by Complete and Nonparticipant-Seen Groups*

| Use of Clinic: Proportion of Total In-Community Time | Complete | | Nonparticipant | |
|---|---|---|---|---|
| | *N* | Per Cent | *N* | Per Cent |
| None | 23 | 25 | 29 | 55 |
| Less than half | 22 | 24 | 10 | 19 |
| Half to nearly all | 15 | 16 | 4 | 8 |
| All | 31 | 34 | 10 | 19 |
| Total | 91 | ∻100 | 53 | ∻100 |

$\chi^2 = 13.21, p < .005$

*Table N-6. Use of Spring Grove State Hospital Outpatient Clinic during Posthospital Year as Related to Type of Release in Complete and Nonparticipant-Seen Groups*

| Use of Clinic | Type of Release | | | | | |
|---|---|---|---|---|---|---|
| | Convalescent Leave | | Discharge | | Total | |
| | *N* | Per Cent | *N* | Per Cent | *N* | Per Cent |
| Complete ($p < .05$): | | | | | | |
| Did not use clinic | 17 | 21 | 6 | 55 | 23 | 25 |
| Used clinic | 63 | 79 | 5 | 45 | 68 | 75 |
| Total | 80 | 100 | 11 | 100 | 91 | 100 |
| Nonparticipant ($p < .001$): | | | | | | |
| Did not use clinic | 15 | 39 | 14 | 93 | 29 | 55 |
| Used clinic | 23 | 61 | 1 | 7 | 24 | 45 |
| Total | 38 | 100 | 15 | 100 | 53 | 100 |

*Table N-7. Use of Spring Grove Outpatient Clinic during Posthospital Year by Complete and Nonparticipant-Seen Groups, Analyzed Separately for Convalescent Leave Patients and Discharged Patients*

| Use of Clinic: Proportion of Total In-Community Time | Complete | | Nonparticipant | |
|---|---|---|---|---|
| | *N* | Per Cent | *N* | Per Cent |
| Convalescent leave only ($p < .05$): | | | | |
| None | 17 | 21 | 15 | 39 |
| Some or all | 63 | 79 | 23 | 61 |
| Total | 80 | 100 | 38 | 100 |
| Discharged only ($p < .10$): | | | | |
| None | 6 | 55 | 14 | 93 |
| Some or all | 5 | 45 | 1 | 7 |
| Total | 11 | 100 | 15 | 100 |

ported, between the two groups (Table N-5). Step 2 was to determine, within each of the two groups separately, whether or not type of release made a difference as to treatment participation (Table N-6). In this instance the answer was affirmative. In Step 3, by rearranging the same data, we controlled for type of release and ascertained whether or not completes and nonparticipant-seens still differed significantly (Table N-7). Again for this variable the answer was mainly affirmative—significantly so within the more numerous convalescent leave group, and near-significantly within the discharged group.

Three other treatment variables showed essentially this same pattern of results—viz., differences persisting even with type of release controlled: (1) proportion of Month-1 time during which drug was used; (2) proportion of total in-community time during which drug was used; and (3) typical daily drug consumption during Month 1.

Five other treatment variables, when analyzed as in Step 2, showed nonsignificant results—thus leaving Step 3 unnecessary, and leaving intact the complete-*vs.*-nonparticipant-seen differences. They were: (1) total number of outpatient facilities used during the year; (2) treatment by a nonpsychiatric physician during the year; and (3) drug usage as measured by (a) proportion of time during latest in-community month, (b) typical daily dosage during latest in-community month, and (c) maximum typical daily consumption at any time.

Only two treatment variables, among the ten which had suggested sampling bias, failed to show persisting significant differences when type of release was controlled. They were (1) use of Spring Grove Outpatient Clinic during Months 1 and/or 12, and (2) treatment by nonpsychiatric physician during Months 1 and/or 12.

### *Effect of Interview Time Lag on Nonparticipant-Seens' Reports*

We have already raised the issue of possible differential distortion of condensed interview reports as a function of time interval between the end of the posthospital year and the date of the interview. To test for such effects, we analyzed nine of the variables on which significant results had suggested sampling bias. The nine were chosen as those for which we were largely unable to verify interview reports, and which seemed most vulnerable to retrospective distortion.

The nonparticipant-seens were subdivided into two (or where possible, three) subgroups differing as to amount of time lag. For six of the nine condensed interview variables tested, variation in the reported information as a function of time lag was negligible: The lowest $p$ value was .30 and the remainder ranged from .50 to .95. The six variables in question were (1) female homemaker responsibility at Month 1; (2) total number of treatment facilities used during the year; and drug usage as indicated by (3) proportion of time during latest in-community month, (4) proportion of all in-community time, (5) typical daily dosage during latest in-community month, and (6) minimum typical daily dosage at any time. On the remaining three variables, *longer* time lag was associated with *more* reported drug usage, with one of the three chi squares yielding borderline significance. All of these pertained to drug usage: (1) proportion of time during Month 1, $p < .005$; (2) typical daily dosage during Month 1, $p < .01$; and (3) maximum typical daily dosage at any time, $p < .10$.

Retrospective distortion, aggravated by time lag, thus appears to have affected some but certainly not all of the nonparticipant study findings. Interestingly enough, on the three variables where distortion did seem present, its direction was consistenly such as would have *attenuated* the observed significant differences between completes and nonparticipant-seens. The fact that those differences did nevertheless emerge, plus the predominance of *nonsignificant* time-lag effects in the total of nine variables analyzed, suggests that the lag effect per se has not seriously occluded any real differences between completes and nonparticipant-seens. Moreover, the pattern of results in these nine analyses suggests distinctly that the lag-distortion was limited largely if not entirely to those few items which pertained only to Month 1 (the point furthest back in time) and which called for highly specific information, e.g., the amount of medication consumed.

APPENDIX N

# DIFFERENCES AMONG COMPLETES, SEMICOMPLETES, AND INCOMPLETES

To whatever extent our three *participant* data groups are dissimilar, one must again allow for sampling bias in interpreting results—especially the study's prime findings, i.e., those based on the 91 complete cases. We have therefore undertaken some strategic comparisons among the three participant data-groups—aimed as before at specifying the nature and extent of sampling bias.

## *Course of Adjustment: Rehospitalization*

Gross differences as to rehospitalization for the study year as a whole are depicted in the chapter on Course of Adjustment, where they are seen to be nonsignificant (Tables III-1 and III-2). Two finer-grained analyses, taking into account monthly rates, are presented in Table N-8. Tabulated percentages are based on subgroup totals: 2 per cent of the 91 completes were "in hospital" at Month 1, and so on. From the monthly significance tests it is clear that, especially during the midyear months 4 through 9, completes were "in hospital" more frequently than semicompletes and incompletes, and that they likewise led in cumulative percentage "rehospitalized first time." Semicompletes and incompletes did not differ consistently from each other at successive months. At the anchor months 1 and 12, on which many of our substantive analyses are based, there were no pronounced hospitalization differences among any of the three subgroups.

## *Background Variables*

Type of release was the only 1 of our 12 background variables on which differences approached the .05 level of significance. As shown in Table N-9, completes tended somewhat more often to be on convalescent leave instead of direct discharge. Sex and number of children were the next most nearly significant discriminating items. For most of the other nine background variables, significance levels were greater than .70.

*Table N-8. Monthly Differences among Complete, Semicomplete, and Incomplete Groups on Hospital Confinement (Noncumulative) and Rehospitalization (Cumulative)*

| Rehospitalization Status | Per Cent, $(p)$[a] | | | | | | | | | | | |
|---|---|---|---|---|---|---|---|---|---|---|---|---|
| | Month 1 | 2 | 3 | 4 | 5 | 6 | 7 | 8 | 9 | 10 | 11 | 12 |
| In hospital (noncumulative): | | | | | | | | | | | | |
| Complete ($N$ = 91) | 2 | 12 | 13 | 14 | 15 | 20 | 23 | 29 | 30 | 24 | 22 | 24 |
| Semicomplete ($N$ = 29) | 7 | 10 | 10 | 3 | 3 | 0 | 3 | 7 | 7 | 14 | 14 | 14 |
| Incomplete ($N$ = 19) | 0 | 0 | 0 | 0 | 5 | 11 | 5 | 11 | 21 | 21 | 11 | 16 |
| All patients ($N$ = 139)[b] | 2.9 | 10.1 | 10.8 | 10.1 | 11.5 | 14.4 | 16.6 | 21.6 | 23.7 | 21.6 | 18.7 | 20.9 |
| $p$[a] | | (.02) | | (.05) | (.05) | (.02) | (.005) | (.025) | (.05) | | | |
| Rehospitalized first time (cumulative): | | | | | | | | | | | | |
| Complete ($N$ = 91) | 2 | 12 | 13 | 19 | 22 | 26 | 31 | 36 | 38 | 40 | 42 | 44 |
| Semicomplete ($N$ = 29) | 7 | 10 | 10 | 10 | 14 | 14 | 17 | 17 | 17 | 21 | 21 | 24 |
| Incomplete ($N$ = 19) | 0 | 0 | 0 | 0 | 5 | 10 | 10 | 16 | 21 | 21 | 21 | 26 |
| All patients ($N$ = 139)[b] | 2.9 | 10.1 | 10.8 | 14.4 | 18.0 | 21.6 | 25.2 | 29.5 | 31.7 | 33.1 | 34.5 | 37.4 |
| $p$[a] | | | | (.05) | (.10) | | (.10) | (.10) | (.10) | (.10) | (.05) | (.10) |

[a]Based on chi square tests; $p$ values greater than .10 are not shown. Small cell frequencies precluded both of the chi square tests for Month 1 and, for "in hospital," required pooling of semicomplete and incomplete frequencies at Months 2 to 7.

[b]These rates are graphed in Fig. III-1.

*Table N-9. Background Variables Showing Greatest Differences among Complete, Semicomplete, and Incomplete Groups*

| Item | Complete | | Semicomplete | | Incomplete | | Total | |
|---|---|---|---|---|---|---|---|---|
| | *N* | Per Cent | *N* | Per Cent | *N* | Per Cent | *N* | Per Cent |
| Sex ($p < .25$): | | | | | | | | |
| Male | 25 | 27 | 13 | 45 | 6 | 32 | 44 | 31.7 |
| Female | 66 | 73 | 16 | 55 | 13 | 68 | 95 | 68.3 |
| Number of children ($p < .20$): | | | | | | | | |
| None | 22 | 24 | 5 | 17 | 9 | 47 | 36 | 25.9 |
| One or two | 38 | 42 | 15 | 52 | 6 | 32 | 59 | 42.4 |
| Three or more | 31 | 34 | 9 | 31 | 4 | 21 | 44 | 31.7 |
| Type of release ($p < .10$): | | | | | | | | |
| Convalescent leave | 80 | 88 | 21 | 72 | 14 | 74 | 115 | 82.7 |
| Discharge | 11 | 12 | 8 | 28 | 5 | 26 | 24 | 17.3 |

## *Adjustment at Months 1 and 12*

On all 26 adjustment variables, data-group differences were tested by *F* at Month 1 and by *t* at Month 12 (Tables N-10 and N-11). (*N*s at Month 12 are reduced by missing scores on all incompletes and on hospitalized completes and semicompletes.) Except on those variables tabulated, no differences reached the .10

*Table N-10. Adjustment Variables Showing Greatest Differences among Complete, Semicomplete, and Incomplete Groups at Month 1*

| Item | Mean, (S. D.) | | | |
|---|---|---|---|---|
| | Complete ($N = 91$) | Semicomplete ($N = 29$) | Incomplete ($N = 19$) | All Participants ($N = 139$) |
| Patient KAS: | | | | |
| *Sym* ($p < .05$) | 22.6* (19.5) | 18.3 (14.8) | 10.5 (13.8) | 20.1 (18.4) |
| *SSA* ($p < .025$) | 9.2* (8.9) | 6.5 (7.6) | 3.8 (3.5) | 7.9 (8.4) |
| Informant KAS: | | | | |
| *FTA* ($p < .01$) | 49.9* (4.8) | 49.6 (5.3) | 45.6 (6.5) | 49.2 (5.4) |
| Stress Index: | | | | |
| *Str-I* ($p < .05$) | 17.5 (14.0) | 17.9* (14.9) | 7.9 (11.5) | 16.3 (14.3) |

*Worst mean score on each variable.

*Table N-11. Adjustment Variables Showing Greatest Differences between Complete and Semicomplete Groups at Month 12*

| Item | Mean, (S. D.) | | | | | |
|---|---|---|---|---|---|---|
| | Complete ($N$ = 69) | | Semicomplete ($N$ = 25) | | Both Groups ($N$ = 94) | |
| Patient KAS: | | | | | | |
| *SEA* ($p<.10$) | 36.5 | (5.2) | 34.2* | (4.9) | 35.9 | (5.2) |
| *LOE* ($p<.05$) | 38.2 | (5.0) | 35.8* | (5.0) | 37.5 | (5.2) |
| *FTA* ($p<.10$) | 46.8 | (7.7) | 50.1* | (5.4) | 47.6 | (7.3) |

*Worst mean score on each variable.

level, and nearly all showed $F$ and $t$ values close to pure chance expectations.

## *Life Situation at Months 1 and 12*

Tests for possible sampling bias in reference to the 40 life-situation variables were handled in the same manner as for adjustment variables, i.e., Months 1 and 12 were analyzed across the board. Significant discriminations ($p < .05$) were found on only two variables at Month 1 and five at Month 12. They are shown in Tables N-12 and N-13, along with several others which most nearly approached significance. Here again, overall results show negligible evidence of any serious sampling bias, and hence do not merit extended discussion. Of passing interest is the tendency, among the stress items at Month 1, for semicompletes to show highest positive frequencies and incompletes lowest; the same holds for the single significant stress item at Month 12.

*Table N-12. Life-Situation Variables Showing Greatest Differences among Complete, Semicomplete, and Incomplete Groups at Month 1*

| Item | Respondent | Complete | | Semicomplete | | Incomplete | | Total | |
|---|---|---|---|---|---|---|---|---|---|
| | | *N* | Per Cent | *N* | Per Cent | *N* | Per Cent | *N* | Per Cent |
| Treatment | | | | | | | | | |
| Drug: how long prescribed ($p < .20$):[a] | Informant | | | | | | | | |
| None or part of month | | 15 | 17 | 4 | 14 | 6 | 33 | 25 | 18.4 |
| All month | | 74 | 83 | 25 | 86 | 12 | 67 | 111 | 81.6 |
| Stress | | | | | | | | | |
| General: "Good" event(s) ($p < .20$): | Informant | | | | | | | | |
| None | | 44 | 48 | 11 | 38 | 13 | 68 | 68 | 48.9 |
| Some | | 47 | 52 | 18 | 62 | 6 | 32 | 71 | 51.1 |
| General: "Bad" event(s) ($p < .05$): | Informant | | | | | | | | |
| Some | | 36 | 40 | 15 | 52 | 3 | 16 | 54 | 38.8 |
| None | | 55 | 60 | 14 | 48 | 16 | 84 | 85 | 61.2 |
| Interpersonal stress ($p < .10$): | Informant | | | | | | | | |
| Some | | 36 | 40 | 14 | 48 | 3 | 16 | 53 | 38.1 |
| None | | 55 | 60 | 15 | 52 | 16 | 84 | 86 | 61.9 |
| Marital and sexual stress ($p < .10$): | Informant | | | | | | | | |
| Some | | 22 | 24 | 11 | 38 | 2 | 11 | 35 | 25.2 |
| None | | 69 | 76 | 18 | 62 | 17 | 89 | 104 | 74.8 |
| Economic and domestic stress ($p < .10$): | Patient | | | | | | | | |
| Some | | 27 | 30 | 12 | 41 | 2 | 11 | 41 | 29.5 |
| None | | 64 | 70 | 17 | 59 | 17 | 89 | 98 | 70.5 |
| Economic and domestic stress ($p < .02$): | Informant | | | | | | | | |
| Some | | 37 | 41 | 9 | 31 | 1 | 5 | 47 | 33.8 |
| None | | 54 | 59 | 20 | 69 | 18 | 95 | 92 | 66.2 |

[a]All $p$ values based on $\chi^2$. Some cases excluded from "drug: how long prescribed" tabulation; see Appendix R.

*Table N-13. Life-Situation Variables Showing Greatest Differences between Complete and Semicomplete Groups at Month 12*

| Item | Respondent | Complete | | Semicomplete | | Total | |
|---|---|---|---|---|---|---|---|
| | | *N* | Per Cent | *N* | Per Cent | *N* | Per Cent |
| Home and Family | | | | | | | |
| Type of Home ($p < .025$):[a] | Patient | | | | | | |
| Conjugal | | 51 | 74 | 12 | 48 | 63 | 67 |
| Parental | | 7 | 10 | 7 | 28 | 14 | 15 |
| All other | | 11 | 16 | 6 | 24 | 17 | 18 |
| Own children away from home ($p < .20$): | Patient | | | | | | |
| None | | 38 | 55 | 12 | 48 | 50 | 53 |
| One | | 19 | 28 | 4 | 16 | 23 | 24 |
| Two to eight | | 12 | 17 | 9 | 36 | 21 | 22 |
| Closest living relative ($p < .05$): | Patient | | | | | | |
| Spouse | | 57 | 83 | 15 | 60 | 72 | 77 |
| Parent, child, or sibling | | 12 | 17 | 10 | 40 | 22 | 23 |
| Informant ($p < .05$): | Informant | | | | | | |
| Spouse | | 40 | 58 | 9 | 36 | 49 | 52 |
| Parent | | 7 | 10 | 8 | 32 | 15 | 16 |
| Son or daughter | | 8 | 12 | 1 | 4 | 9 | 10 |
| Sibling | | 6 | 9 | 4 | 16 | 10 | 11 |
| All other | | 8 | 12 | 3 | 12 | 11 | 12 |

| | | | | | | | |
|---|---|---|---|---|---|---|---|
| Treatment | | | | | | | |
| Where received ($p < .05$): | Patient | | | | | | |
| Nowhere | | 18 | 26 | 10 | 40 | 28 | 30 |
| Spring Grove Outpatient Clinic | | 29 | 42 | 7 | 28 | 36 | 38 |
| Public clinic other than Spring Grove | | 10 | 14 | 0 | 0 | 10 | 11 |
| All other | | 12 | 17 | 8 | 32 | 20 | 21 |
| Stress | | | | | | | |
| Physical health ($p < .01$): | Informant | | | | | | |
| Some | | 12 | 17 | 12 | 48 | 24 | 26 |
| None | | 57 | 83 | 13 | 52 | 70 | 74 |

[a]All $p$ values based on $\chi^2$. In some of the tests, adjacent cells were pooled to meet minimum frequency requirements.

Appendix O

# *Procedure for Calculating KAS Global Adjustment Score

The KAS global adjustment score is a combination of five weighted KAS raw scores. It was originally developed in an earlier follow-up study of 75 patients who had lived in the community for about one year after leaving Spring Grove State Hospital. As empirically derived, it constituted an optimum estimate (from concurrent KAS scores) of a competent clinical rating of the patient's global in-community adjustment.

The criterion was a single comprehensive rating of "general clinical condition and overall functioning," made jointly by an experienced clinical psychologist who interviewed the patient and an experienced social worker who interviewed an informant. Neither interviewer had access to the KAS scores which were obtained on the same day. The criterion rating was scaled as follows:

7 The patient's overall condition, taking into account his functioning in the clinical, social, and occupational areas, is comparable to the upper 20 per cent of ex-hospitalized patients; his overall functioning is as good as or better than that of the average person in the community.

6 The patient's overall functioning is comparable to that of the upper 20 per cent of ex-hospitalized patients, but is not as good as that of the average person in the community.

5 The patient's overall functioning is above average for ex-hospitalized patients.

4 The patient's overall functioning is about average for ex-hospitalized patients.

3 The patient's overall functioning is below average for ex-hospitalized patients.

2 The patient's overall functioning is comparable to that of the lower 20 per cent of ex-hospitalized patients, but he does not require hospitalization.

1 The patient's overall functioning is extremely poor, patient would be ranked in the lower 20 per cent of ex-hospitalized patients; patient should be hospitalized and would be except for the presence of very favorable social circumstances.

The Summerfield and Lubin (1951) method of selecting a minimum set of predictors was used in analyzing the regression of the 24 KAS scores on the criterion. Five KAS scores proved optimally combinable for estimating the clinicians' adjustment rating, yielding a multiple *r* of .83.

Raw scores in the formula are:

$Y$ = Global Adjustment Rating
$X_1$ = KAS S2, Level of Performance of Socially-Expected Activities (patient's report)
$X_2$ = KAS R2, Level of Performance of Socially-Expected Activities (informant's report)
$X_3$ = KAS S3, Level of Expectations (patient's report)
$X_4$ = KAS R1 Cluster 9, Nervousness
$X_5$ = KAS R1 Cluster 11, Bizarreness

The multiple regression formula is:

$$Y = -.386 + .195\,X_1 + .068\,X_2 - .070\,X_3 - .114\,X_4 - .176\,X_5$$

Note that the direction of the global adjustment scale is opposite to that of most KAS raw scores, i.e., high global scores favorable and low scores unfavorable.

Appendix P

# Gross Content Classification of the 26 Adjustment Variables

To aid in interpreting results throughout the report, we have adopted a three-way classification of the 26 adjustment variables. The grouping is based essentially on manifest item content. Class 1, psychopathological, contains the measures dealing with "negative mental health," i.e., direct manifestations of illness in the form of symptoms or disturbed behavior. (The stress index is included in Class 1 on grounds of the hypothetical relationship: stress, to stress reaction, to symptoms or disturbed behavior.) Class 2, social, deals with "positive mental health" as reflected in constructive role-taking and wholesome use of free time. Class 3, judgmental, contains those scales in which the patient's behavior in the social area (Class 2) is being appraised—either by himself or by his informant, and either directly or (as in the discrepancy measures, *SSA-P* and *SSA-I*) indirectly.

| KAS Form No. | Title | Symbol | Respondent |
|---|---|---|---|
| | *Class 1: Psychopathological (16 variables)* | | |
| S1 | Symptom Discomfort | *Sym* | Patient |
| R1 (1) | Belligerence | *Bel* | Informant |
| R1 (2) | Verbal Expansiveness | *Exp* | Informant |

| KAS Form No. | Title | Symbol | Respondent |
|---|---|---|---|
| R1 (3) | Negativism | *Neg* | Informant |
| R1 (4) | Helplessness | *Hel* | Informant |
| R1 (5) | Suspiciousness | *Sus* | Informant |
| R1 (6) | Anxiety | *Anx* | Informant |
| R1 (7) | Withdrawal and Retardation | *Wdl* | Informant |
| R1 (8) | General Psychopathology | *Psy* | Informant |
| R1 (9) | Nervousness | *Ner* | Informant |
| R1 (10) | Confusion | *Con* | Informant |
| R1 (11) | Bizarreness | *Biz* | Informant |
| R1 (12) | Hyperactivity | *Hyp* | Informant |
| R1 (13) | Emotional Stability | *Sta* | Informant |
| – | Stress Index | *Str-P* | Patient |
| – | Stress Index | *Str-I* | Informant |
| | *Class 2: Social (4 variables)* | | |
| S2 | Level of Performance of Socially-Expected Activities | *SEA-P* | Patient |
| R2 | Level of Performance of Socially-Expected Activities | *SEA-I* | Informant |
| RS4 | Level of Free-Time Activities | *FTA-P* | Patient |
| RS4 | Level of Free-Time Activities | *FTA-I* | Informant |
| | *Class 3: Judgmental (6 variables)* | | |
| S3 | Level of Expectations | *LOE-P* | Patient |
| R3 | Level of Expectations | *LOE-I* | Informant |
| S2, S3 | Level of Satisfaction with Performance of Socially-Expected Activities | *SSA-P*<br>*SSA-P* | Patient<br>Patient |
| R2, R3 | Level of Satisfaction with Performance of Socially-Expected Activities | *SSA-I* | Informant |
| S5 | Level of Satisfaction with Free-Time Activities | *SFA-P* | Patient |
| R5 | Level of Satisfaction with Free-Time Activities | *SFA-I* | Informant |

Appendix Q

# *Procedure for Calculating KAS Outcome Index

The outcome index can be used in any research where a single score is needed to indicate net change from initial to later or final observation. In our study, the initial and final observations in question were the KAS global adjustment scores (Appendix O) for Months 1 and 12.

Statistically, the outcome index is a refinement of the usual change score, initial minus final. It takes into account individual differences in initial scores, and the index of change is a standard score, not a raw score.

---

*Step 1.* Find the range of initial raw scores.

Example: range = 7 to 116 for hypothetical array of scores.

*Step 2.* Tabulate frequency ($f$) distribution of initial raw scores ($X$), and pool adjacent class intervals as needed to form Groups large enough to analyze separately in succeeding Steps.

Example:

| $X$ | $f$ | Group |
|---|---|---|
| 107-116 | 1 | |
| 97-106 | 1 | |
| 87-96 | 1 | I |
| 77-86 | 3 | |
| 67-76 | 2 | |
| 57-66 | 20 | II |
| 47-56 | 22 | III |
| 37-46 | 45 | IV |
| 27-36 | 46 | V |
| 17-26 | 25 | VI |
| 7-16 | 4 | |

*Step 3.* For each Group separately, compile initial and final raw scores ($X$, $Y$) and compute change scores ($X - Y = C$).

Example (Group I):

| $X$ | $Y$ | $C$ |
|---|---|---|
| 116 | 27 | 89 |
| 91 | 26 | 65 |
| 97 | 23 | 74 |
| 80 | 80 | 0 |
| 82 | 42 | 40 |
| 69 | 23 | 46 |
| 73 | 21 | 52 |
| 77 | 13 | 64 |

*Step 4.* Compute mean ($M$) and standard deviation ($\sigma$) of change scores for each Group.

Example (Group I):

$M_{C_I} = 53.75$

$\sigma_{C_I} = 25.06$

*Step 5.* Compute outcome index ($Z$) for each subject by the formula:

$$Z = \frac{C - M_C}{\sigma_C} \times 100 + 500$$

Example (Group I, $C = 89$):

$$Z = \frac{89 - 53.75}{25.06} \times 100 + 500 = 640.66$$

Appendix R

# *Explanations of Missing Data on 10 Life-Situation Items

In analyzing and reporting the life-situation interview information, we have routinely excluded data falling in the familiar categories "does not apply" and "unknown." Such exclusions occur in many of the tabulations throughout the report; "does not apply" omissions are generally much more numerous than "unknown."

To avoid needless repetition in footnotes, Table R-1 presents complete explanations of all exclusions.

*Table R-1. Cases Excluded from Life-Situation Data Analyses*

| Item | Respondent | Item No.[a] | Cases Excluded |
|---|---|---|---|
| Work and Homemaking | | | |
| Busiest single work week | Patient | 19 | Unemployed patients |
| Busiest single work week | Informant | 6 | Unemployed patients; or employed, but informant does not know answer |
| Breadwinner contribution | Informant | 7 | Patients with no dependents to support |
| Homemaker responsibility | Patient | 17 | Male patients |
| Homemaker responsibility | Informant | 4 | Male patients |
| Treatment | | | |
| Drug: how long prescribed | Informant | 1 | Informant does not know |
| Drug use: duration | Patient | 6 | Patients with no drug prescribed |

*(Table R-1, continued)*

| Item | Respondent | Item No.[a] | Cases Excluded |
|---|---|---|---|
| Drug use: duration | Informant | 2 | Patients with no drug prescribed; or drug prescribed, but informant does not know answer |
| Drug use: daily amount | Patient | 7 | Patients with no drug prescribed |
| Drug use: daily amount | Informant | 3 | Patients with no drug prescribed; or drug prescribed, but informant does not know answer |

[a]As shown in interview form for patient (Appendix H) or informant (Appendix I).

Appendix S

# Monthly Results from Trend Analysis of Complete Nonrelapser Group

The following table supplements our textual presentation of the trend analysis results by providing complete summary information on all 26 adjustment variables.

*Table S-1. Adjustment Variables: Monthly Means (Upper Row) and Standard Deviations (Lower Row) from 12-Month Trend Analysis (Complete Nonrelapsers, N = 51)*

| Variable | Month 1 | 2 | 3 | 4 | 5 | 6 | 7 | 8 | 9 | 10 | 11 | 12 |
|---|---|---|---|---|---|---|---|---|---|---|---|---|
| Patient KAS | | | | | | | | | | | | |
| *Sym* | 22.7 | 22.4 | 18.3 | 18.4 | 16.9 | 17.5 | 16.4 | 19.1 | 17.3 | 15.4 | 14.2 | 13.2 |
| | 19.5 | 21.2 | 17.2 | 18.1 | 17.4 | 21.1 | 20.6 | 20.5 | 19.7 | 19.1 | 17.4 | 17.7 |
| *SEA-P* | 36.4 | 35.4 | 36.3 | 36.3 | 37.1 | 36.8 | 36.6 | 36.8 | 37.0 | 37.1 | 37.1 | 37.4 |
| | 5.3 | 5.6 | 5.2 | 4.9 | 4.7 | 4.7 | 5.2 | 5.1 | 4.8 | 5.4 | 5.2 | 5.0 |
| *LOE-P* | 37.3 | 38.2 | 39.1 | 39.0 | 38.2 | 39.0 | 38.8 | 38.5 | 38.9 | 38.6 | 38.4 | 38.5 |
| | 4.6 | 5.1 | 5.1 | 5.0 | 5.0 | 5.1 | 4.7 | 5.0 | 5.3 | 5.7 | 5.6 | 5.4 |
| *SSA-P* | 7.5 | 10.0 | 8.5 | 8.6 | 6.7 | 7.3 | 7.8 | 6.2 | 6.5 | 5.6 | 5.4 | 6.0 |
| | 7.8 | 10.0 | 9.7 | 8.5 | 6.7 | 7.0 | 8.8 | 6.2 | 6.1 | 6.9 | 6.2 | 7.0 |
| *FTA-P* | 47.6 | 48.4 | 47.7 | 47.3 | 47.4 | 47.4 | 46.5 | 47.9 | 47.0 | 47.7 | 46.9 | 46.8 |
| | 5.5 | 5.9 | 6.3 | 5.6 | 6.0 | 6.4 | 6.4 | 6.0 | 7.3 | 6.3 | 7.3 | 7.3 |
| *SFA-P* | 29.9 | 30.4 | 28.6 | 29.0 | 28.2 | 29.2 | 28.5 | 28.2 | 28.3 | 28.0 | 28.5 | 27.6 |
| | 5.7 | 7.3 | 6.8 | 6.7 | 5.0 | 5.8 | 5.5 | 5.4 | 5.2 | 6.4 | 5.7 | 5.6 |

*(Table S-1, continued)*

| Variable | Month 1 | 2 | 3 | 4 | 5 | 6 | 7 | 8 | 9 | 10 | 11 | 12 |
|---|---|---|---|---|---|---|---|---|---|---|---|---|
| Informant KAS R1 | | | | | | | | | | | | |
| *Bel* | 4.5 | 4.5 | 4.5 | 4.4 | 4.4 | 4.3 | 4.2 | 4.2 | 4.3 | 4.3 | 4.4 | 4.4 |
| | 0.9 | 0.8 | 0.8 | 0.8 | 0.8 | 0.8 | 0.6 | 0.4 | 0.8 | 0.7 | 0.9 | 0.9 |
| *Exp* | 6.2 | 5.8 | 6.1 | 5.9 | 6.0 | 6.0 | 5.9 | 5.8 | 5.9 | 5.9 | 6.1 | 6.1 |
| | 2.3 | 1.7 | 2.1 | 2.1 | 2.2 | 2.0 | 2.0 | 2.1 | 1.9 | 2.0 | 2.4 | 2.2 |
| *Neg* | 12.1 | 11.5 | 11.8 | 11.6 | 11.4 | 11.3 | 10.9 | 11.0 | 11.1 | 11.0 | 11.4 | 11.1 |
| | 2.7 | 2.3 | 3.2 | 2.8 | 2.8 | 2.9 | 2.6 | 2.7 | 2.6 | 3.1 | 3.2 | 2.7 |
| *Hel* | 5.7 | 5.2 | 5.4 | 5.4 | 5.4 | 5.1 | 5.0 | 5.1 | 4.8 | 5.0 | 4.9 | 5.0 |
| | 1.8 | 1.6 | 1.8 | 1.8 | 1.9 | 1.5 | 1.5 | 1.7 | 1.3 | 1.6 | 1.7 | 1.5 |
| *Sus* | 4.9 | 4.8 | 4.8 | 4.7 | 4.5 | 4.5 | 4.3 | 4.4 | 4.3 | 4.3 | 4.4 | 4.6 |
| | 1.6 | 1.4 | 1.4 | 1.4 | 1.2 | 1.2 | 0.7 | 1.0 | 0.7 | 0.8 | 0.9 | 1.3 |
| *Anx* | 7.7 | 6.7 | 7.1 | 7.0 | 6.8 | 6.7 | 6.4 | 6.6 | 6.5 | 6.5 | 6.5 | 6.4 |
| | 2.6 | 1.7 | 2.1 | 2.4 | 1.9 | 1.6 | 1.2 | 1.6 | 1.3 | 1.7 | 1.6 | 1.0 |
| *Wdl* | 9.4 | 9.2 | 9.3 | 9.3 | 9.1 | 9.0 | 8.7 | 8.3 | 8.4 | 8.4 | 8.4 | 8.3 |
| | 2.4 | 3.0 | 3.3 | 3.4 | 3.7 | 3.7 | 3.0 | 2.6 | 2.9 | 2.9 | 3.3 | 3.1 |
| *Psy* | 33.8 | 32.5 | 32.8 | 32.1 | 31.7 | 31.3 | 30.1 | 30.7 | 30.0 | 30.6 | 30.8 | 30.5 |
| | 7.0 | 7.2 | 7.9 | 7.8 | 8.3 | 7.4 | 6.9 | 7.4 | 7.2 | 7.8 | 8.8 | 8.2 |
| *Ner* | 7.6 | 6.8 | 6.8 | 6.8 | 6.6 | 6.8 | 6.3 | 6.4 | 6.5 | 6.4 | 6.3 | 6.1 |
| | 2.3 | 2.1 | 2.5 | 2.5 | 2.6 | 2.5 | 2.3 | 2.5 | 2.3 | 2.3 | 2.5 | 2.3 |
| *Con* | 3.4 | 3.1 | 3.1 | 3.1 | 3.2 | 3.1 | 3.2 | 3.1 | 3.0 | 3.1 | 3.1 | 3.3 |
| | 1.3 | 0.3 | 0.2 | 0.4 | 0.8 | 0.5 | 0.7 | 0.6 | 0.1 | 0.4 | 0.3 | 1.2 |
| *Biz* | 5.7 | 5.6 | 5.5 | 5.6 | 5.5 | 5.5 | 5.4 | 5.6 | 5.5 | 5.5 | 5.6 | 5.6 |
| | 1.2 | 1.1 | 1.1 | 1.1 | 1.2 | 1.1 | 0.9 | 1.2 | 0.9 | 0.8 | 1.1 | 1.1 |
| *Hyp* | 4.7 | 4.1 | 4.1 | 4.2 | 3.9 | 3.9 | 3.9 | 3.7 | 3.8 | 3.8 | 3.9 | 3.7 |
| | 1.3 | 1.1 | 1.4 | 1.6 | 1.3 | 1.2 | 1.1 | 1.1 | 1.0 | 1.2 | 1.2 | 1.3 |
| *Sta* | 30.5 | 30.6 | 30.4 | 30.7 | 30.9 | 30.8 | 31.0 | 31.7 | 31.9 | 31.5 | 31.2 | 30.9 |
| | 4.2 | 4.5 | 5.0 | 5.8 | 5.2 | 5.2 | 5.2 | 4.6 | 5.0 | 5.4 | 5.3 | 5.5 |
| Informant KAS R2 to 5 | | | | | | | | | | | | |
| *SEA-I* | 35.5 | 35.6 | 36.0 | 36.3 | 36.6 | 36.7 | 36.8 | 37.1 | 37.3 | 37.1 | 36.9 | 36.7 |
| | 4.6 | 5.1 | 4.5 | 5.1 | 5.1 | 5.5 | 5.2 | 5.5 | 5.6 | 5.6 | 5.7 | 5.3 |
| *LOE-I* | 34.3 | 35.5 | 36.7 | 37.3 | 37.5 | 37.0 | 37.9 | 38.1 | 38.1 | 37.8 | 38.1 | 37.6 |
| | 5.0 | 4.8 | 5.3 | 4.7 | 5.1 | 4.9 | 5.4 | 5.5 | 5.1 | 5.0 | 4.9 | 4.9 |
| *SSA-I* | 4.6 | 6.1 | 6.0 | 6.8 | 6.1 | 5.9 | 5.8 | 6.2 | 5.9 | 5.9 | 7.3 | 6.3 |
| | 5.9 | 6.9 | 6.9 | 7.4 | 6.6 | 7.0 | 6.7 | 7.2 | 6.6 | 7.6 | 8.5 | 7.6 |
| *FTA-I* | 49.1 | 48.2 | 48.2 | 48.0 | 47.5 | 47.5 | 47.4 | 46.9 | 46.5 | 47.4 | 47.3 | 47.9 |
| | 4.6 | 5.8 | 5.8 | 6.0 | 6.2 | 6.7 | 6.5 | 6.4 | 7.3 | 7.3 | 6.9 | 7.0 |
| *SFA-I* | 28.8 | 27.8 | 27.6 | 28.4 | 27.1 | 27.5 | 27.2 | 27.1 | 26.4 | 26.8 | 26.9 | 26.2 |
| | 4.3 | 4.6 | 5.1 | 5.6 | 4.9 | 5.1 | 4.6 | 5.2 | 4.5 | 5.6 | 4.7 | 4.5 |

*(Table S-1, continued)*

| Variable | Month 1 | 2 | 3 | 4 | 5 | 6 | 7 | 8 | 9 | 10 | 11 | 12 |
|---|---|---|---|---|---|---|---|---|---|---|---|---|
| Stress | | | | | | | | | | | | |
| *Str-P* | 15.5 | 16.4 | 14.6 | 15.7 | 13.9 | 14.8 | 14.6 | 15.6 | 12.0 | 10.4 | 12.1 | 12.4 |
| | 13.5 | 13.9 | 13.8 | 14.8 | 13.4 | 12.7 | 13.4 | 13.5 | 12.2 | 11.8 | 12.6 | 11.1 |
| *Str-I* | 17.3 | 15.5 | 15.3 | 15.5 | 13.9 | 14.0 | 12.2 | 12.9 | 11.2 | 12.7 | 10.2 | 12.2 |
| | 13.9 | 12.6 | 15.3 | 13.6 | 13.6 | 14.4 | 13.0 | 12.9 | 11.8 | 11.0 | 11.0 | 11.5 |

Appendix T

# *T* Score Conversions for the Katz Adjustment Scales

As a by-product of our monthly KAS administrations, we developed *T* scores based on the group of 51 complete nonrelapsers. Tables T-1 and T-2 present the KAS raw-to-*T* score conversions for tests administered at posthospital Months 1 and 12.

As a normative group, the sample is of course considerably smaller than desirable, though it has the compensating advantage of having been carefully selected, described, and studied. The most relevant information about these patients is presented in Chapter III; see Tables III-11 and III-12 for description in terms of background variables.

If used with appropriate caution, the *T* scores should prove helpful not only to researchers but also to clinicians evaluating individual cases by means of the KAS. On suitably calibrated graph paper, the clinician can plot individual KAS profiles which will be analogous (though not normatively comparable) to the familiar Minnesota Multiphasic Personality Inventory profile. In general, *T* scores below average (50) will reflect comparatively good adjustment; those patients who can be maintained with minimal treatment or who may not need treatment will usually be found in this range. Conversely, *T* scores well above 50 will suggest a need for relatively close clinical attention. (The scales measuring satisfaction and expectation–those which we classify as judgmental in

Appendix P—will of course not serve as direct measures of disturbance, but can provide guidelines for counseling with patients and informants.)

Several points must be kept clearly in mind if misuse of *T* scores is to be avoided. Foremost is the nature of the norm group: These are patients of the white race whose clinical and environmental conditions enabled them to remain unrehospitalized for at least one year following treatment in a large state mental institution. Most of them received outpatient aftercare with drugs during the posthospital period.

A special caution applies to the Month-12 *T* scores. The patients on whom these norms are based had typically completed 11 previous KAS testings at monthly intervals. If these *T* scores are used with a patient who has taken the KAS for the first time, for instance, it is likely that test-retest effects peculiar to the norm group will penalize the newly tested patient by way of slight spurious elevation of his KAS profile.

Two final constraints apply only to the KAS *Sym* (Symptom Discomfort) score. (1) Any obtained raw score on this scale must be reduced by 55 before entering the raw score column of Table T-1 or T-2; this is necessary in order to match the corresponding adjustments we have made in processing *Sym* raw scores in the present study (Table II-3, footnote b). (2) The maximum possible raw score on *Sym*, after this correction is made, is 165; however, 99 is the highest raw score listed in the conversion tables. (No adjusted raw score higher than 99 was involved in developing these norms; to have listed higher scores would have unduly stretched the upper ends of the two tables.) For obtained raw scores higher than 99, at five-point intervals, *T* score conversions for Months 1 and 12 respectively are as follows (in parentheses): 100 (90, 99), 105 (92, 102), 110 (95, 105), 115 (97, 107), 120 (100, 110), 125 (102, 113), 130 (105, 116), 135 (108, 119), 140 (110, 122), 145 (113, 124), 150 (115, 127), 155 (118, 130), 160 (120, 133), 165 (123, 136).

# APPENDIX T

*Table T-1. T Score Conversions for the 24 Katz Adjustment Scales: First Posthospital Month*

| Raw Score | Patient KAS | | | | | | Informant KAS R1 | | | | | | | | | | | | | Informant KAS R2 to 5 | | | | |
|---|---|---|---|---|---|---|---|---|---|---|---|---|---|---|---|---|---|---|---|---|---|---|---|---|
| | *Sym* | *SEA-P* | *LOE-P* | *SSA-P* | *FTA-P* | *SFA-P* | *Bel* | *Exp* | *Neg* | *Hel* | *Sus* | *Anx* | *Wdl* | *Psy* | *Ner* | *Con* | *Biz* | *Hyp* | *Sta* | *SEA-I* | *LOE-I* | *SSA-I* | *FTA-I* | *SFA-I* |
| 99 | 90 | | | | | | | | | | | | | | | | | | | | | | | |
| 98 | 89 | | | | | | | | | | | | | | | | | | | | | | | |
| 97 | 89 | | | | | | | | | | | | | | | | | | | | | | | |
| 96 | 88 | | | | | | | | | | | | | 140 | | | | | | | | | | |
| 95 | 87 | | | | | | | | | | | | | 139 | | | | | | | | | | |
| 94 | 87 | | | | | | | | | | | | | 137 | | | | | | | | | | |
| 93 | 86 | | | | | | | | | | | | | 136 | | | | | | | | | | |
| 92 | 86 | | | | | | | | | | | | | 134 | | | | | | | | | | |
| 91 | 85 | | | | | | | | | | | | | 133 | | | | | | | | | | |
| 90 | 85 | | | | | | | | | | | | | 131 | | | | | | | | | | |
| 89 | 84 | | | | | | | | | | | | | 130 | | | | | | | | | | |
| 88 | 84 | | | | | | | | | | | | | 128 | | | | | | | | | | |
| 87 | 83 | | | | | | | | | | | | | 127 | | | | | | | | | | |
| 86 | 83 | | | | | | | | | | | | | 126 | | | | | | | | | | |
| 85 | 82 | | | | | | | | | | | | | 124 | | | | | | | | | | |
| 84 | 82 | | | | | | | | | | | | | 123 | | | | | | | | | | |
| 83 | 81 | | | | | | | | | | | | | 121 | | | | | | | | | | |
| 82 | 81 | | | | | | | | | | | | | 120 | | | | | | | | | | |
| 81 | 80 | | | | | | | | | | | | | 118 | | | | | | | | | | |
| 80 | 80 | | | | | | | | | | | | | 117 | | | | | | | | | | |
| 79 | 79 | | | | | | | | | | | | | 115 | | | | | | | | | | |
| 78 | 79 | | | | | | | | | | | | | 114 | | | | | | | | | | |
| 77 | 78 | | | | | | | | | | | | | 113 | | | | | | | | | | |
| 76 | 78 | | | | | | | | | | | | | 111 | | | | | | | | | | |
| 75 | 77 | | | | | | | | | | | | | 110 | | | | | | | | | | |
| 74 | 77 | | | | | | | | | | | | | 108 | | | | | | | | | | |
| 73 | 76 | | | | | | | | | | | | | 107 | | | | | | | | | | |
| 72 | 76 | | | | | | | | | | | | | 105 | | | | | | | | | | |
| 71 | 75 | | | | | | | | | | | | | 104 | | | | | | | | | | |
| 70 | 75 | | | | | | | | | | | | | 102 | | | | | | | | | | |
| 69 | 74 | | | | | | | | | | | | | 101 | | | | | | | | | | |
| 68 | 73 | | | | | | | | | | | | | 100 | | | | | | | | | | |
| 67 | 73 | | | 127 | | | | | | | | | | 98 | | | | | | | | 156 | | |
| 66 | 72 | | | 126 | 83 | 114 | | | | | | | | 97 | | | | | | | | 155 | 87 | 137 |
| 65 | 72 | | | 125 | 82 | 112 | | | | | | | | 95 | | | | | | | | 153 | 85 | 135 |
| 64 | 71 | | | 124 | 80 | 111 | | | | | | | | 94 | | | | | | | | 151 | 83 | 133 |
| 63 | 71 | | | 122 | 78 | 109 | | | | | | | | 92 | | | | | | | | 150 | 81 | 130 |
| 62 | 70 | | | 121 | 76 | 107 | | | | | | | | 91 | | | | | | | | 148 | 78 | 128 |
| 61 | 70 | | | 120 | 74 | 105 | | | | | | | | 89 | | | | | | | | 146 | 76 | 126 |

# APPENDIX T

| | | | | | | | | | | | | | | | | | | | | | | |
|---|---|---|---|---|---|---|---|---|---|---|---|---|---|---|---|---|---|---|---|---|---|---|
| 60 | 69 | | | 118 | 73 | 103 | | | | | | | | 88 | | | | | | 144 | 74 | 123 |
| 59 | 69 | | | 117 | 71 | 102 | | | | | | | | 86 | | | | | | 143 | 72 | 121 |
| 58 | 68 | | | 116 | 69 | 100 | | | | | | | | 85 | | | | | | 141 | 70 | 119 |
| 57 | 68 | | | 114 | 67 | 98 | | | | | | | | 84 | | | | | | 139 | 67 | 116 |
| 56 | 67 | | | 113 | 65 | 96 | | | | | | | | 82 | | | | | | 138 | 65 | 114 |
| 55 | 67 | | | 112 | 63 | 95 | | | | | | | | 81 | | | | | | 136 | 63 | 112 |
| 54 | 66 | | | 111 | 62 | 93 | | | | | | | | 79 | | | | | | 134 | 61 | 109 |
| 53 | 66 | | | 109 | 60 | 91 | | | | | | | | 78 | | | | | | 133 | 59 | 107 |
| 52 | 65 | | | 108 | 58 | 89 | | | | | | | | 76 | | | | | | 131 | 56 | 105 |
| 51 | 65 | | | 107 | 56 | 88 | | | | | | | | 75 | | | | | | 129 | 54 | 102 |
| 50 | 64 | | | 105 | 54 | 86 | | | | | | | | 73 | | | | | | 127 | 52 | 100 |
| 49 | 64 | | | 104 | 52 | 84 | | | | | | | | 72 | | | | | | 126 | 50 | 98 |
| 48 | 63 | 28 | 26 | 103 | 51 | 82 | | | | | | | | 71 | | | | 23 | 22 | 124 | 48 | 95 |
| 47 | 63 | 30 | 28 | 101 | 50 | 80 | | | | | | | | 69 | | | | 25 | 24 | 122 | 45 | 93 |
| 46 | 62 | 32 | 31 | 100 | 47 | 79 | | | | | | | | 68 | | | | 27 | 26 | 121 | 43 | 90 |
| 45 | 62 | 33 | 33 | 99 | 45 | 77 | | | | | | | | 66 | | | | 29 | 28 | 119 | 41 | 88 |
| 44 | 61 | 35 | 35 | 98 | 43 | 75 | | | | | | | | 65 | | | | 31 | 30 | 117 | 39 | 86 |
| 43 | 61 | 47 | 37 | 96 | 42 | 73 | | | | | | | | 63 | | | | 34 | 32 | 115 | 37 | 83 |
| 42 | 60 | 39 | 39 | 95 | 40 | 72 | | | | | | | | 62 | | | | 36 | 34 | 114 | 35 | 81 |
| 41 | 59 | 41 | 42 | 94 | 38 | 70 | | | | | | | | 60 | | | | 38 | 37 | 112 | 32 | 79 |
| 40 | 59 | 43 | 44 | 92 | 36 | 68 | | | | | | | | 59 | | | | 40 | 39 | 110 | 30 | 76 |
| 39 | 58 | 45 | 46 | 91 | 34 | 66 | | | | | | | | 58 | | | | 42 | 41 | 109 | 28 | 74 |
| 38 | 58 | 47 | 48 | 90 | 32 | 64 | | | | | | | | 56 | | | | 45 | 43 | 107 | 26 | 72 |
| 37 | 57 | 49 | 50 | 88 | 31 | 63 | | | | | | | | 55 | | | | 47 | 45 | 105 | 24 | 69 |
| 36 | 57 | 51 | 53 | 87 | 29 | 61 | | | 140 | | | | | 53 | | | 37 | 49 | 47 | 103 | 21 | 67 |
| 35 | 56 | 53 | 55 | 86 | 27 | 59 | | | 136 | | | | | 52 | | | 39 | 50 | 49 | 102 | 19 | 65 |
| 34 | 56 | 54 | 57 | 84 | 25 | 57 | | | 133 | | | | | 50 | | | 42 | 53 | 50 | 100 | 17 | 62 |
| 33 | 55 | 56 | 59 | 83 | 23 | 56 | | | 129 | | | | | 50 | | | 44 | 55 | 53 | 98 | 15 | 60 |
| 32 | 55 | 58 | 62 | 82 | 21 | 54 | | | 125 | | | | | 47 | | | 46 | 58 | 55 | 97 | 13 | 58 |
| 31 | 54 | 60 | 64 | 81 | 20 | 52 | | | 121 | | | | | 46 | | | 49 | 60 | 57 | 95 | 10 | 55 |
| 30 | 54 | 62 | 66 | 79 | 18 | 50 | | | 118 | | | | | 45 | | | 50 | 62 | 59 | 93 | 8 | 53 |
| 29 | 53 | 64 | 68 | 78 | 16 | 48 | | | 114 | | | | | 43 | | | 54 | 64 | 61 | 92 | 6 | 51 |
| 28 | 53 | 66 | 70 | 77 | 14 | 47 | | | 110 | | | | | 42 | | | 56 | 66 | 63 | 90 | 4 | 48 |
| 27 | 52 | 68 | 73 | 75 | 12 | 45 | | | 106 | | | | | 40 | | | 58 | 69 | 65 | 88 | 2 | 46 |
| 26 | 52 | 70 | 75 | 74 | 10 | 43 | | | 103 | | | | | 39 | | | 61 | 71 | 67 | 86 | | 44 |
| 25 | 51 | 72 | 77 | 73 | 9 | 41 | | | 99 | | | | | 37 | | | 63 | 73 | 69 | 85 | | 41 |
| 24 | 51 | 74 | 79 | 71 | 7 | 40 | | | 95 | | | 112 | 112 | 36 | | | 66 | 75 | 71 | 83 | | 39 |
| 23 | 50 | 76 | 82 | 70 | 5 | 38 | | | 91 | | | 109 | 108 | | | | 68 | 77 | 73 | 81 | | 36 |
| 22 | 50 | 78 | 84 | 69 | 3 | 36 | | | 87 | | | 105 | 104 | | | | 71 | 79 | 75 | 80 | | 34 |
| 21 | 50 | 79 | 86 | 68 | | | | | 84 | | | 101 | 99 | | | | 73 | 82 | 77 | 78 | | |
| 20 | 50 | 81 | 88 | 66 | | | | 111 | 80 | | | 97 | 95 | | | 167 | 75 | 84 | 79 | 76 | | |
| 19 | 48 | 83 | 90 | 65 | | | | 106 | 76 | | | 93 | 91 | | | 158 | 78 | 86 | 81 | 74 | | |
| 18 | 48 | 85 | 93 | 64 | | | | 102 | 72 | | | 90 | 87 | | | 150 | 80 | 88 | 83 | 73 | | |
| 17 | 47 | 87 | 95 | 62 | | | | 98 | 69 | | | 86 | 82 | | | 142 | 83 | 90 | 85 | 71 | | |
| 16 | 47 | 89 | 97 | 61 | | | 179 | 93 | 65 | 108 | 121 | 82 | 78 | | 87 | 134 | 85 | 93 | 87 | 69 | | |

*(Table T-1, continued)*

| Raw Score | Patient KAS | | | | | | Informant KAS R1 | | | | | | | | | | | | | Informant KAS R2 to 5 | | | | |
|---|---|---|---|---|---|---|---|---|---|---|---|---|---|---|---|---|---|---|---|---|---|---|---|---|
| | *Sym* | *SEA-P* | *LOE-P* | *SSA-P* | *FTA-P* | *SFA-P* | *Bel* | *Exp* | *Neg* | *Hel* | *Sus* | *Anx* | *Wdl* | *Psy* | *Ner* | *Con* | *Biz* | *Hyp* | *Sta* | *SEA-I* | *LOE-I* | *SSA-I* | *FTA-I* | *SFA-I* |
| 15 | 46 | | | 60 | | | 168 | 89 | 61 | 103 | 115 | 78 | 74 | | 83 | | 126 | | 88 | | | 68 | | |
| 14 | 45 | | | 58 | | | 156 | 84 | 57 | 97 | 109 | 74 | 70 | | 78 | | 118 | | 90 | | | 66 | | |
| 13 | 45 | | | 57 | | | 145 | 80 | 53 | 91 | 102 | 70 | 65 | | 74 | | 110 | | 92 | | | 64 | | |
| 12 | 44 | | | 56 | | | 134 | 76 | 50 | 86 | 96 | 67 | 61 | | 69 | 117 | 101 | 105 | 95 | | | 63 | | |
| 11 | 44 | | | 55 | | | 123 | 71 | 46 | 80 | 89 | 63 | 57 | | 65 | 109 | 93 | 97 | 97 | | | 61 | | |
| 10 | 43 | | | 53 | | | 111 | 67 | 42 | 74 | 83 | 59 | 53 | | 60 | 101 | 85 | 90 | 100 | | | 59 | | |
| 9 | 43 | | | 52 | | | 100 | 62 | 38 | 69 | 77 | 55 | 48 | | 56 | 93 | 77 | 82 | 102 | | | 57 | | |
| 8 | 42 | | | 51 | | | 89 | 58 | | 63 | 70 | 51 | 44 | | 52 | 86 | 69 | 75 | | | | 56 | | |
| 7 | 42 | | | 50 | | | 78 | 54 | | 57 | 64 | 47 | 40 | | 47 | 78 | 61 | 67 | | | | 54 | | |
| 6 | 41 | | | 48 | | | 67 | 50 | | 52 | 57 | 44 | 36 | | 43 | 70 | 53 | 60 | | | | 52 | | |
| 5 | 41 | | | 47 | | | 55 | 45 | | 46 | 51 | | | | 38 | 62 | 45 | 52 | | | | 51 | | |
| 4 | 40 | | | 45 | | | 44 | | | 40 | 44 | | | | 34 | 55 | | 45 | | | | 50 | | |
| 3 | 40 | | | 44 | | | | | | | | | | | | 47 | | 37 | | | | 47 | | |
| 2 | 39 | | | 43 | | | | | | | | | | | | | | | | | | 45 | | |
| 1 | 39 | | | 42 | | | | | | | | | | | | | | | | | | 44 | | |
| 0 | 38 | | | 40 | | | | | | | | | | | | | | | | | | 42 | | |

# APPENDIX T

*Table T-2. T Score Conversions for the 24 Katz Adjustment Scales: 12th Posthospital Month*

| Raw Score | Patient KAS | | | | | | Informant KAS R1 | | | | | | | | | | | | | Informant KAS R2 to 5 | | | | |
|---|---|---|---|---|---|---|---|---|---|---|---|---|---|---|---|---|---|---|---|---|---|---|---|---|
| | *Sym* | *SEA-P* | *LOE-P* | *SSA-P* | *FTA-P* | *SFA-P* | *Bel* | *Exp* | *Neg* | *Hel* | *Sus* | *Anx* | *Wdl* | *Psy* | *Ner* | *Con* | *Biz* | *Hyp* | *Sta* | *SEA-I* | *LOE-I* | *SSA-I* | *FTA-I* | *SFA-I* |
| 99 | 99 | | | | | | | | | | | | | | | | | | | | | | | |
| 98 | 98 | | | | | | | | | | | | | | | | | | | | | | | |
| 97 | 98 | | | | | | | | | | | | | | | | | | | | | | | |
| 96 | 97 | | | | | | | | | | | | | 131 | | | | | | | | | | |
| 95 | 97 | | | | | | | | | | | | | 130 | | | | | | | | | | |
| 94 | 96 | | | | | | | | | | | | | 129 | | | | | | | | | | |
| 93 | 95 | | | | | | | | | | | | | 127 | | | | | | | | | | |
| 92 | 95 | | | | | | | | | | | | | 126 | | | | | | | | | | |
| 91 | 94 | | | | | | | | | | | | | 125 | | | | | | | | | | |
| 90 | 94 | | | | | | | | | | | | | 124 | | | | | | | | | | |
| 89 | 93 | | | | | | | | | | | | | 122 | | | | | | | | | | |
| 88 | 93 | | | | | | | | | | | | | 121 | | | | | | | | | | |
| 87 | 92 | | | | | | | | | | | | | 120 | | | | | | | | | | |
| 86 | 91 | | | | | | | | | | | | | 119 | | | | | | | | | | |
| 85 | 91 | | | | | | | | | | | | | 117 | | | | | | | | | | |
| 84 | 90 | | | | | | | | | | | | | 116 | | | | | | | | | | |
| 83 | 90 | | | | | | | | | | | | | 115 | | | | | | | | | | |
| 82 | 89 | | | | | | | | | | | | | 114 | | | | | | | | | | |
| 81 | 89 | | | | | | | | | | | | | 112 | | | | | | | | | | |
| 80 | 88 | | | | | | | | | | | | | 111 | | | | | | | | | | |
| 79 | 87 | | | | | | | | | | | | | 110 | | | | | | | | | | |
| 78 | 87 | | | | | | | | | | | | | 109 | | | | | | | | | | |
| 77 | 86 | | | | | | | | | | | | | 108 | | | | | | | | | | |
| 76 | 86 | | | | | | | | | | | | | 106 | | | | | | | | | | |
| 75 | 85 | | | | | | | | | | | | | 105 | | | | | | | | | | |
| 74 | 85 | | | | | | | | | | | | | 104 | | | | | | | | | | |
| 73 | 84 | | | | | | | | | | | | | 103 | | | | | | | | | | |
| 72 | 83 | | | | | | | | | | | | | 101 | | | | | | | | | | |
| 71 | 83 | | | | | | | | | | | | | 100 | | | | | | | | | | |
| 70 | 82 | | | | | | | | | | | | | 99 | | | | | | | | | | |
| 69 | 82 | | | | | | | | | | | | | 98 | | | | | | | | | | |
| 68 | 81 | | | | | | | | | | | | | 96 | | | | | | | | | | |
| 67 | 81 | | | 138 | | | | | | | | | | 95 | | | | | | | | 130 | | |
| 66 | 80 | | | 136 | 77 | 119 | | | | | | | | 94 | | | | | | | | 129 | 76 | 139 |
| 65 | 79 | | | 135 | 75 | 117 | | | | | | | | 93 | | | | | | | | 128 | 75 | 137 |
| 64 | 79 | | | 133 | 74 | 115 | | | | | | | | 91 | | | | | | | | 126 | 73 | 134 |
| 63 | 78 | | | 132 | 72 | 113 | | | | | | | | 90 | | | | | | | | 125 | 72 | 132 |
| 62 | 78 | | | 130 | 71 | 112 | | | | | | | | 89 | | | | | | | | 124 | 70 | 130 |
| 61 | 77 | | | 129 | 70 | 110 | | | | | | | | 88 | | | | | | | | 122 | 69 | 128 |

*(Table T-2, continued)*

| Raw Score | Patient KAS Sym | SEA-P | LOE-P | SSA-P | FTA-P | SFA-P | Informant KAS R1 Bel | Exp | Neg | Hel | Sus | Anx | Wdl | Psy | Ner | Con | Biz | Hyp | Sta | Informant KAS R2 to 5 SEA-I | LOE-I | SSA-I | FTA-I | SFA-I |
|---|---|---|---|---|---|---|---|---|---|---|---|---|---|---|---|---|---|---|---|---|---|---|---|---|
| 60 | 77 | | | 127 | 68 | 108 | | | | | | | | 86 | | | | | | | | 121 | 68 | 125 |
| 59 | 76 | | | 126 | 67 | 106 | | | | | | | | 85 | | | | | | | | 120 | 66 | 123 |
| 58 | 76 | | | 125 | 65 | 104 | | | | | | | | 84 | | | | | | | | 118 | 65 | 121 |
| 57 | 75 | | | 123 | 64 | 103 | | | | | | | | 83 | | | | | | | | 117 | 63 | 119 |
| 56 | 74 | | | 122 | 63 | 101 | | | | | | | | 82 | | | | | | | | 116 | 62 | 116 |
| 55 | 74 | | | 120 | 61 | 99 | | | | | | | | 80 | | | | | | | | 114 | 60 | 114 |
| 54 | 73 | | | 119 | 60 | 97 | | | | | | | | 79 | | | | | | | | 113 | 59 | 112 |
| 53 | 73 | | | 117 | 59 | 95 | | | | | | | | 78 | | | | | | | | 112 | 57 | 110 |
| 52 | 72 | | | 116 | 57 | 94 | | | | | | | | 77 | | | | | | | | 110 | 56 | 108 |
| 51 | 72 | | | 115 | 56 | 92 | | | | | | | | 75 | | | | | | | | 109 | 55 | 105 |
| 50 | 71 | | | 113 | 54 | 90 | | | | | | | | 74 | | | | | | | | 108 | 53 | 103 |
| 49 | 70 | | | 112 | 53 | 88 | | | | | | | | 73 | | | | | | | | 106 | 52 | 101 |
| 48 | 70 | 28 | 32 | 110 | 52 | 86 | | | | | | | | 72 | | | | | | 28 | 28 | 105 | 50 | 99 |
| 47 | 69 | 31 | 34 | 109 | 50 | 85 | | | | | | | | 70 | | | | | | 30 | 31 | 104 | 50 | 96 |
| 46 | 69 | 33 | 36 | 107 | 50 | 83 | | | | | | | | 69 | | | | | | 32 | 33 | 103 | 47 | 94 |
| 45 | 68 | 35 | 38 | 106 | 47 | 81 | | | | | | | | 68 | | | | | | 34 | 35 | 101 | 46 | 92 |
| 44 | 68 | 37 | 40 | 105 | 46 | 79 | | | | | | | | 67 | | | | | | 36 | 37 | 100 | 44 | 90 |
| 43 | 67 | 39 | 42 | 103 | 45 | 78 | | | | | | | | 65 | | | | | | 38 | 39 | 99 | 43 | 87 |
| 42 | 66 | 41 | 43 | 102 | 43 | 76 | | | | | | | | 64 | | | | | | 40 | 41 | 97 | 42 | 85 |
| 41 | 66 | 43 | 45 | 100 | 42 | 74 | | | | | | | | 63 | | | | | | 42 | 43 | 96 | 40 | 83 |
| 40 | 65 | 45 | 47 | 99 | 41 | 72 | | | | | | | | 62 | | | | | | 44 | 45 | 95 | 39 | 81 |
| 39 | 65 | 47 | 49 | 97 | 39 | 70 | | | | | | | | 60 | | | | | | 46 | 47 | 93 | 37 | 78 |
| 38 | 64 | 49 | 50 | 96 | 38 | 69 | | | | | | | | 59 | | | | | | 47 | 49 | 92 | 36 | 76 |
| 37 | 64 | 50 | 53 | 94 | 36 | 67 | | | | | | | | 58 | | | | | | 49 | 50 | 91 | 34 | 74 |
| 36 | 63 | 53 | 55 | 93 | 35 | 65 | | | 141 | | | | | 57 | | | | | 41 | 50 | 53 | 89 | 33 | 72 |
| 35 | 62 | 55 | 57 | 92 | 34 | 63 | | | 138 | | | | | 56 | | | | | 42 | 53 | 56 | 88 | 31 | 70 |
| 34 | 62 | 57 | 59 | 90 | 32 | 61 | | | 134 | | | | | 54 | | | | | 44 | 55 | 58 | 87 | 30 | 67 |
| 33 | 61 | 59 | 60 | 89 | 31 | 60 | | | 130 | | | | | 53 | | | | | 46 | 57 | 60 | 85 | 28 | 65 |
| 32 | 61 | 61 | 62 | 87 | 29 | 58 | | | 127 | | | | | 52 | | | | | 48 | 59 | 62 | 84 | 27 | 63 |
| 31 | 60 | 63 | 64 | 86 | 28 | 56 | | | 123 | | | | | 51 | | | | | 50 | 61 | 64 | 83 | 26 | 61 |
| 30 | 60 | 65 | 66 | 84 | 27 | 54 | | | 119 | | | | | 50 | | | | | 52 | 63 | 66 | 81 | 24 | 58 |
| 29 | 59 | 67 | 68 | 83 | 25 | 52 | | | 116 | | | | | 48 | | | | | 54 | 65 | 68 | 80 | 23 | 56 |
| 28 | 58 | 69 | 70 | 82 | 24 | 51 | | | 112 | | | | | 47 | | | | | 55 | 66 | 70 | 79 | 21 | 54 |
| 27 | 58 | 71 | 72 | 80 | 23 | 50 | | | 108 | | | | | 46 | | | | | 57 | 68 | 72 | 77 | 20 | 52 |
| 26 | 57 | 73 | 74 | 79 | 21 | 47 | | | 105 | | | | | 44 | | | | | 59 | 70 | 74 | 76 | 18 | 50 |
| 25 | 57 | 75 | 76 | 77 | 20 | 45 | | | 101 | | | | | 43 | | | | | 61 | 72 | 76 | 75 | 17 | 47 |
| 24 | 56 | 77 | 77 | 76 | 18 | 44 | | | 97 | | | 221 | 102 | 42 | | | | | 63 | 74 | 78 | 73 | 15 | 45 |
| 23 | 56 | 79 | 79 | 74 | 17 | 42 | | | 94 | | | 211 | 98 | | | | | | 65 | 76 | 80 | 72 | 14 | 43 |
| 22 | 55 | 81 | 81 | 73 | 16 | 40 | | | 90 | | | 201 | 95 | | | | | | 67 | 78 | 83 | 71 | 13 | 41 |
| 21 | 54 | 83 | 83 | 72 | | | | | 86 | | | 192 | 92 | | | | | | 68 | 80 | 85 | 69 | | |

# APPENDIX T

| | | | | | | | | | | | | | | | | | | | |
|---|---|---|---|---|---|---|---|---|---|---|---|---|---|---|---|---|---|---|---|
| 20 | 54 | 85 | 85 | 70 | | 115 | 83 | | | 182 | 89 | | | 185 | | 70 | 82 | 87 | 68 |
| 19 | 53 | 87 | 87 | 69 | | 110 | 79 | | | 172 | 85 | | | 176 | | 72 | 84 | 89 | 67 |
| 18 | 53 | 89 | 89 | 67 | | 106 | 75 | | | 163 | 82 | | | 166 | | 74 | 85 | 91 | 65 |
| 17 | 52 | 91 | 91 | 66 | | 101 | 72 | | | 153 | 79 | | | 157 | | 76 | 87 | 93 | 64 |
| 16 | 52 | 94 | 93 | 64 | 180 | 96 | 68 | 125 | 135 | 143 | 75 | 93 | | 147 | | 78 | 89 | 95 | 63 |
| 15 | 51 | | | 63 | 169 | 92 | 64 | 118 | 128 | 133 | 72 | 89 | | 138 | | 79 | | | 61 |
| 14 | 50 | | | 61 | 158 | 87 | 61 | 111 | 120 | 124 | 69 | 84 | | 129 | | 81 | | | 60 |
| 13 | 50 | | | 60 | 147 | 82 | 57 | 105 | 113 | 114 | 65 | 80 | | 119 | | 83 | | | 59 |
| 12 | 50 | | | 59 | 135 | 78 | 53 | 98 | 105 | 104 | 62 | 76 | 121 | 110 | 116 | 85 | | | 58 |
| 11 | 50 | | | 57 | 124 | 73 | 50 | 91 | 98 | 95 | 59 | 71 | 113 | 101 | 108 | 87 | | | 56 |
| 10 | 48 | | | 56 | 113 | 68 | 46 | 84 | 90 | 85 | 56 | 67 | 104 | 91 | 100 | 89 | | | 55 |
| 9 | 48 | | | 54 | 102 | 64 | 42 | 77 | 83 | 75 | 52 | 63 | 96 | 82 | 92 | 91 | | | 54 |
| 8 | 47 | | | 53 | 90 | 59 | | 71 | 75 | 65 | 50 | 58 | 88 | 73 | 84 | | | | 52 |
| 7 | 46 | | | 51 | 79 | 54 | | 64 | 68 | 56 | 46 | 54 | 80 | 63 | 76 | | | | 51 |
| 6 | 46 | | | 50 | 68 | 50 | | 57 | 60 | 46 | 42 | 50 | 72 | 54 | 68 | | | | 50 |
| 5 | 45 | | | 50 | 57 | 45 | | 50 | 53 | | | 45 | 64 | 45 | 60 | | | | 48 |
| 4 | 45 | | | 47 | 45 | | | 43 | 45 | | | 41 | 56 | | 52 | | | | 47 |
| 3 | 44 | | | 46 | | | | | | | | | 47 | | 45 | | | | 46 |
| 2 | 44 | | | 44 | | | | | | | | | | | | | | | 44 |
| 1 | 43 | | | 43 | | | | | | | | | | | | | | | 43 |
| 0 | 42 | | | 41 | | | | | | | | | | | | | | | 42 |

Appendix U

# Afterthoughts on Administration, Method, Examiners, and Respondents

The natural history of any research project abounds with workaday circumstances and experiences which rarely find their way into reports of results. Some of those elements are scientifically extraneous and hence are rightfully omitted. But others, if reflected upon, reveal potential value either for thorough understanding of results or for planning and conducting further investigations in the same or related areas.

In its nature and execution, our project was by way of being unusual and improbable. In a sense, these qualities will appear less prominent when clinical and psychosocial research has moved more decisively into the areas of community mental health and aftercare. Meanwhile, for what it can be worth to those who spearhead that movement, we shall here augment previous comments on salient features of the project's method and execution. We shall largely avoid mention of what is general or elementary in doing research, as well as what is too specific or ephemeral to be useful to others; and we shall ignore those big things that made little difference.

Three conditions of the project have much to do with what is to be gleaned from our experience. (1) It had a year-long study period requiring frequently repeated contact between examiners and respondents and eliciting of sensitive personal information.

(2) Participation by patients and informants was altogether voluntary—not bound or predisposed by any concurrent linkages with treatment, employment, residence, or the like. (3) The prime subjects had psychiatric illnesses of varying kinds and severity, for which they had recently received inpatient treatment.

---

## *THE PROJECT'S ADMINISTRATIVE AND PROFESSIONAL MILIEU

A clinical research team usually stands in some quite particular relation to at least one treatment facility, and that relation must pervasively influence its operations. Our treatment facility, Spring Grove State Hospital, has been described in Chapter I; we have also mentioned its Outpatient Clinic, located on the hospital grounds, where we were able to test many of our subjects in conjunction with their aftercare appointments. Beginning in 1953 with a small professional and clerical cadre, the Spring Grove Research Department had in the sixties attained a diversified maturity. While project data were being collected, numerous other staff members were pursuing studies in chemotherapy, neurophysiology, biochemistry, psychological measurement, and neo-Pavlovian salivary conditioning in humans.

Although the Research Department was officially based at the hospital, the hospital did not fully encompass it either geographically, operationally, or fiscally. Financial support for research came not only from the State of Maryland but also from U.S. Public Health Service grants, from manufacturers of psychotropic drugs, and from a few other sources. Most of the department's business was managed by an unusual local nonprofit corporation named Friends of Psychiatric Research, Inc. Among the self-delegated purposes of "Friends" were to promote research interest and participation among laymen and the public in general, to raise money for research, and to relieve professional research personnel of distracting administrative chores. The last-named function, much to be valued, spared us countless hours of nonscientific but necessary work—in procuring supplies and services, in preparing nontechnical reports and correspondence, and in negotiating policy and practical arrangements with hospital officials.

With the hospital, the Research Department's day-to-day working relationship was one of productive but not uncomplicated coexistence. At all levels, frictions between the two parallel organizations were neither more nor less abrasive than could be expected and tolerated by a researcher of average worldly wisdom. We experienced a fair share of fluctuation between tranquility and crisis, between peaceful symbiosis and discordant interchange. Adverse phases of the cycle seemed often to involve the garden variety of service-vs.-research antipathy, so amply documented by Kandel and Williams (1964, pp. 35-68). When a hospital clerical official complained acerbically to the Project Director about a study staff worker who had held one of her file cards in his mouth while searching patient records, the usefulness of the Director's clinical training took on an extra dimension. But other circumstances more than compensated for mishaps such as these. For example, our unrestricted access to treatment records on our patients, both in the hospital and in its Outpatient Clinic, not only included charge-out privileges but was greatly facilitated by the spontaneous helpfulness of hospital clerical personnel in charge—a blessing that should never be taken for granted (Kandel and Williams, 1964, pp. 106-107).

Access to treatment records was facilitated also by the project's offices being located in the same building where records were stored and stenographically updated. That location offered several additional logistic advantages. Since it had long been the admission building, all of our patients could more readily find their way to it when they first visited us; moreover, rehospitalized patients were thereby easier to identify and to contact for the relapse test. The fact that the Spring Grove Outpatient Clinic was also situated in our building was likewise advantageous: it simplified not only our use of aftercare records but, more importantly, the combining of testing sessions with treatment visits for those patients who were attending the clinic. The two-in-one appointments were often quite easy to arrange because many patients' clinic visits were, like our tests, scheduled once monthly. We felt that such double-purpose appointments ran less likelihood of being missed;[1] they

[1]The group of 91 complete-data patients contained a larger proportion of persons who had attended the Spring Grove clinic at Month 1 (with or without co-ordinated

also reduced the need for home-visit testing. Another helpful circumstance was that we could be quickly alerted to any subject's rehospitalization whenever it originated in the Spring Grove Outpatient Clinic. Finally, our liaison with the clinic often proved useful for learning patients' current home addresses, both in initial recruiting and in tracing a few persons who moved after having started in the study.

## *SOME FEATURES OF A *MODUS OPERANDI*

It was not by happenstance that we were thus favorably situated. Some of the above advantages had been foreseen when it was decided to station our staff in the admission building. The decision of course had to be approved by hospital authorities; at that time, unlike now, the Research Department had very little space it could call its own. The offices into which we moved had in this instance been previously occupied by the staff of another research project which was nearing completion at the time. Likewise, when our own project finished its data collection and its staff dwindled, we moved to smaller quarters in a comparatively isolated building, there to proceed with data analysis (via a Washington, D.C. computer) and report writing; while our old offices were taken over by a newly nascent investigation. This continuous shifting represented one of several kinds of flexibility that was essential not merely to completing a single project but to a larger scheme of coexistence which had to be acceptable both by a long-established hospital administration and by a rapidly growing league of researchers.

Space for research within the hospital's buildings was by no means plentiful. Ardent bargaining for it was, in fact, the order of the day. Offsetting our own good fortune in that domain was a later round of bargaining which, at the height of our data-collection period, left us suddenly bereft of one of two small but necessary rooms. Both rooms were indispensable to us for testing patients and informants simultaneously and independently; what had made them vulnerable to reallocation was that they were not

testing appointments) than did the semicompletes, and semicompletes contained a larger proportion than incompletes. The trend was in the opposite direction for patients attending other facilities at Month 1, as well as for patients who were untreated at that time. However, the differences were not statistically significant.

continually occupied. Before the problem could be resolved, we had to discontinue recruiting new subjects, notify responsible authorities that the project was thus being delayed, and explain the critical need for the office space in question.

Aside from office space, the most sensitive issue in relations between the project and the hospital was that of confidentiality. It was imperative that we not violate any ex-patient's privilege of concealing the fact of his previous hospitalization. Neither could we allow it to become known to any and all that former inpatients were participating in the study. Thus telephone calls and home visits had to be handled with great delicacy, especially in early overtures when we were unfamiliar with the patient's situation. A green examiner nearly doomed one of our cases when, upon arriving at the patient's home, he proclaimed, "I'm from Spring Grove State Hospital." At one early stage of our operation, procedures for preserving confidentiality in this respect had to be explicitly clarified and guaranteed in a meeting with a key hospital official. Another aspect of the confidentiality problem was entailed in our assurance to each prospective subject that his reports to us would be used only for research (see Appendix B, question 4). Reiteration of this point came to be important for those patients who feared involuntary rehospitalization—an apprehension not without realistic basis in some individuals' previous experience. On the other hand, the hospital was entitled to know of its former patients' participation in our study, and our word-of-mouth co-ordinating actions could not be depended upon to accomplish such notification in every case. Therefore, when each patient completed the study, we routinely entered a note to that effect in his hospital chart. All test and interview data, however, were locked in our research files and were released to others only with the patient's written consent. Only a very few such requests and permissions actually transpired.

Our project's coexistence with and within the hospital would, we believe, have been inordinately difficult, perhaps impossible, if our entire staff had been new to the scene and if the hospital had not itself had considerable prior familiarity with intramural but semi-independent research. As it was, senior project workers were "old hands" at Spring Grove, and so were our three most helpful consultants—a psychiatrist and two social workers. In training newly hired examiners and others, we tried diligently to equip them with their predecessors' knowledge of the hospital's structure, policies, procedures, and personnel. Previous experience in the parent hospital was even valuable in helping us to be more gracious than nonplussed when, as happened more than once, a recently tested patient appeared unannounced in our main office and began dusting and emptying waste baskets. To explain: the patient had been readmitted and had joined the housecleaning crew which always operated not after, but during, office hours!

Not all surprises were that quickly mastered. One day an examiner sat down with a patient, opened his kit, and began explaining the KAS. It was her Month-1 evaluation, and the examiner had not been long on the job. As the test booklet was being shown her, she cut in: "But I just took this test last week!" The examiner, reeling inwardly with wild surmises of errant appointment-making, *déjà vu*, etc., hastily checked the patient's "log notes" (Appendix C)—a standard item always carried in the kit. No previous evaluation was on record. When the dust had cleared, the patient was found to be participating not only in our own study but also in a research evaluation of treatment at a day center she was then attending. No matter; his own double-take now resolved, the examiner helped the patient to resolve hers, and science forged ahead.

Most of what we have further to say about our operating experience can be arranged in readably discrete sections. There are five items, however, which defy neat categorization, having in common only the fact that each proved exceptionally helpful in its own way throughout the project.

1. Private telephone line. Much lost motion was saved by having our own telephone, allocated exclusively to the project and not connected with the hospital switchboard. The Research Department, which had several such phones, found safeguards necessary to prevent their unauthorized after-hours use by persons unknown for long-distance calls.

2. Copying machine. Access to a popular brand of rapid electrostatic copying machine made us wonder how research ever got accomplished without one. For data forms, recurrent messages, etc., the machine eliminated stencil-cutting except for large-

quantity productions such as our life-situation interview booklets. Even more, whenever copies of already existing documents were needed in a hurry, the machine made them readily obtainable.

3. Large wall maps of city and state. The secretary and examiners used our two wall maps daily for locating new subjects' homes and refreshing their memories on the old. We indexed the maps to facilitate this, in manner similar to street-indexing. Patients' typewritten names and addresses were mounted in alphabetical order next to the maps. For each patient, a narrow ribbon was strung from his name to the exact location of his home on the map. We found the system especially useful for newly hired examiners and for co-ordinating appointments so that two or more homes could be visited on a single outbound testing trip. On the state map, an additional logistical aid was a pencil-drawn circle having a radius of 60 miles and with the hospital site in the center. The circle defined the geographical limits of eligibility for the study in terms of place of residence (see Chapter I).

4. Entertainment kit for young children. Some respondents when reporting for tests at our offices would, usually out of necessity, bring with them one or more small children. We kept on hand for them crayons, coloring books, modeling clay, and a few other "quiet hour" playthings. While parents were taking tests, the entertainment kit solaced children, parents, and staff.

5. Literature on methodology and logistics. Some of the best writings we have seen on the matters here under discussion came into print a little too late to be of maximum usefulness to us. Future workers in this field would do well to consult them—*before* planning research studies. Top choices among books are the previously cited volume by Kandel and Williams (1964) and the scholarly handbook on survey research by Hyman (1955). Also worthy of close attention are papers by May, Tuma, and Kraude (1965), by Sargent (1960), and by Williams (1963).

## *PROCEDURAL ISSUES IN SAMPLING AND TESTING

It could be argued that the amount of effort we expended in attempting to obtain a representative sample was wasteful, in view of the fact that what the sample represented was only a single state hospital. From that viewpoint the same effort could be justified only if we had contrived for the sample to represent the average population (as delimited) of *all* state mental hospitals, insofar as possible by examining available statistics. It is certainly true that our findings must not be used as though they applied outright to state hospitals in general, or to any single hospital other than Spring Grove. The other side of the matter is that the project did emphasize the trial demonstration of methods which might prove useful to others, and that, having succeeded reasonably well, we have in this chapter recommended similar studies at the community level wherever they would meet certain needs. From this point of view, if we had sought a nationally representative sample, the study would have resembled a Gallup poll in which respondents, all from within a single city, were so selected as to gauge the opinions of the nation's entire citizenry. In other words, ecological naturalism was for us a higher value than miniaturizing the universal.

There is, however, at least one thing we would handle differently if we had the project to do over again. By hindsight, the sizeable effort involved in establishing liaison with clinics other than Spring Grove's looks to have been misspent. Its purpose, as we have said, was to permit combined testing and treatment appointments for the convenience of those patients who attended the outlying clinics. As it turned out, only a few tests were actually so obtained. Moreover, some clinics required extensive prior documentation concerning examiners, patients, and our research aims and procedures—over and beyond the two-page prospectus which we had routinely provided them to begin with. Nor did the plan appeal even to all of the patients in question; two of them, in fact, objected so seriously that our contact with them in that situation was aborted. Apparently, our effort to combine two appointments in one violated boundaries in their personal schemes of organizing their experience, letting the right hand know what the left was doing.

A different form of co-ordination of research and clinical services was entailed whenever the special relapse test was called for. Now the patient was an inpatient (almost always at Spring Grove), and could be tested only in the hospital setting. We were operating on home ground; ordinarily, the arrangement was smooth and matter-of-fact, though once or twice we ran afoul of hospital administration barriers (Appendix C: notes 3-22, 3-23, and 3-24-65). As was to be expected, the newly readmitted patient's clinical condition also posed testing problems in some cases, necessitating postponement until acute distress or confusion could subside. In only one instance did such a condition persist for so long a time that the relapse test was missed. Informants also had to be seen for relapse tests, often under considerable stress from sharing in the rehospitalization experience. Informant relapse tests proved to be quite manageable nonetheless, and despite the out-of-the-ordinary appointment circumstances. These appointments with informants were of course handled separately from those for the readmitted patients on whom they were reporting. When feasible, we saw the informants as they came to the hospital to visit the patients. Other relapse test appointments for informants followed the usual plan of being completed either by home visit or at our offices.

Another deviation from routine testing procedure was our policy of suspending, until Month 12, efforts to continue evaluating those patients who had missed three or more monthly tests (Figure I-1: box E, steps 8 and 9).[2] When the project was at peak operation with a caseload of about 75, roughly one-fourth of the patients were typically so "suspended," one-fifth were back in the hospital, and the remainder—about 40 individuals—were undergoing monthly evaluations. Those suspended were, by design, all contacted at Month 12 and urged to complete the final test; they had been apprised of our intention to do this at the time they became suspended, and had been asked to promise Test 12 at that juncture. The importance of these suspended cases was that each was destined to become, when closed, either a semicomplete case (Test 12 completed unless patient was back in hospital) or an incomplete case (Test 12 missed). Retrospectively, we still believe that this way of handling attrition among active participants was

[2] For a substantial majority of these renegers, testing efforts were actually interrupted immediately after Test 1—at which point, when we revealed to them our interest in the remaining 11 tests, they demurred. About half of these early renegers, however, were persuaded to complete Test 12.

the method of choice. Two values were involved: conservation of staff time in dealing with renegers, and conservation of usable data.[3]

The surpassing usefulness of the electronic computer in statistical tasks as large as ours goes without saying. Without such equipment our yield of results would have been meager, if indeed the project could have been undertaken at all in anything resembling its accomplished form. Yet, despite the enormous practical importance of computerization for research data of this kind, comment on our own experience in that regard is hardly worth while. Computer technology is advancing so precipitously that whatever we might say on the subject would suffer from built-in obsolescence.

## *TRAVAILS AND PERILS OF EXAMINERS

It would be difficult to overstate the examiners' significance for the success of the project. It began with the recruiting and selection of persons to be so employed. It involved on-the-job training and the management of the examiner's work schedule. In a most crucial sense, it hinged upon each examiner's behavior when, left to his own devices, he sought sensitive and confidential information from unobligated troubled persons and their intimates. A single serious defect in any of the four phases–selection, training, schedule management, job performance–could, if unremedied, have doomed the entire study. We shall limit present comment to schedule management and behavior on the job.

Except during rare slack periods, testing and interviewing were the examiner's sole function, and rightly so. To have assigned him other and unrelated duties would certainly have lowered his effi-

[3]Apropos of the latter criterion, we remain aware that some of the obtained test data were not fully used in this report. For semicomplete cases, analyses were limited largely to Months 1 and 12; for incompletes, to Month 1. Not all of these cases missed all other tests (Figure I-2). But, given the design of the study, there is no discernible major value in these cases' gap-riddled data for Months 2 through 11.

The other segment of unused data is that of the nine relapsers who had not one but two or three rehospitalizations during their posthospital year (Table III-1). We have analyzed data only from their earliest relapse tests, leaving untouched the second and third relapse tests which were also obtained. Here the small number of cases was the chief deterrent, but until the study was finished, we had no sure way of knowing how many such cases there would be.

ciency and threatened to impair his vital professional identification with his mission. Some jobs can suitably be part-time, and the same person can hold more than one of them concurrently; but in intensive psychosocial research, there are very few such positions. We have seen more than one study become painfully impaled on the cavalier transgression of that principle. Fractionated professional identities and shuttlings from one duty to another are not compatible with single-minded immersion in a demanding technical and interpersonal task.

In a sense, the examiner's work was functionally central to the whole project. Its complexities necessitated that other ongoing work be organized supportively around it. A comfortable Monday-through-Friday schedule was out of the question for the examiner: Many appointments for tests had to be on evenings and weekends, with compensatory time off during regular office hours. There were a number of ancillary duties which made the job far more than simply that of psychometrist and interviewer. The examiner drove his private automobile on home visits, recording mileage for reimbursement. He often served as his own secretary when, completing a test, he would make the next monthly appointment and place it on record in the patient's folder. (In this function the project secretary was always "on call" to help him.) Most significantly, in his year-long dealings with patients and informants, he was responsible not only to sustain their interest and cooperativeness, but to share with dignity and meaningful relatedness in the lives of persons who sometimes misperceived him and who often looked to him for help, advice, esteem, vindication, relief of loneliness, and other fulfillments quite foreign to project goals. Not many testing sessions could be terminated directly with completion of the business at hand. A case in point is the one narrated in full in Appendix C; see especially the notes dated 3-15-65 through 3-17-65b. The art of data-gathering demanded that, while responding to each individual as a person—not as a mere object of research—the examiner must become neither aloof nor over-involved. Monthly testing could founder on either extreme. This is not to say, however, that testing was all empathy and altruism. Data being the prime objective, and not a few respondents being reluctant, passively antagonistic, or actively resistant, testing could also have been killed with kindness. The formula for success often required a heady admixture of persuasion, whether in the form of hinting or coaxing, subtle manipulating or firm insistence as appropriate—in principle always benign, and hopefully so in practice. While none of our tactical ingredients are new to the seasoned interview-hunter, in our work they acquired a fourth dimension by virtue of the need for as many as 12 repetitive contacts per subject.

The requirement of strict independence of patient and informant reports, free from collusion and with neither party overhearing the other, seems simple enough. With our two separate testing rooms, its observance was straightforward and routine, but on home visits it could rarely be taken for granted. Here was yet another challenge to the examiner's interpersonal adroitness. When both parties (e. g., husband and wife) were to be tested on a single visit, separateness had to be unofficiously but reliably assured. Only occasionally did the problem loom very large, but it did recur as a complication to be premeditatedly managed.

In Chapter I, we have noted that our standard policy of having the same examiner to serve a given case from start to finish was an unattainable ideal. The extent of deviation from that ideal is manifest in Appendix K: Tables K-5, K-6, and K-7. It took eight separate workers to bring to rest our data collection. (Of these, only five were bona fide examiners; the last three in Table K-5, who participated quite skimpily, were qualified emergency substitutes.) To what extent did examiner-induced variations contaminate our test results? The unresolved state of that question can only be a matter of persisting concern. The "experimenter effect" is an amply documented phenomenon in various research contexts, including projects like our own: "In the area of survey research the phenomenon of modeling has been reported in studies by Cantril . . . and [by] Blankenship . . . who have found that interviewers elicit from their interviewees, at a probability greater than chance, responses which reflect thc interviewers' own beliefs" (Kintz, Delprato, Mettee, Persons, and Schappe, 1965). It is much to be hoped that future investigators will do considerably more about the problem than has been accomplished either by previous workers or by the present paragraph.

# PATIENTS AND INFORMANTS: RESEARCH BEHAVIOR AND MOTIVES

Our year-long relations with patients and informants afforded us a richness of observations and inferences which, as with the psychotherapist, have meanings not bounded by specific service concerns and commitments. Many of those by-products are worth passing on to others. We can only highlight them here; space would permit more, but time does not.

Why did so many subjects *not* elect their rightful option of simply declining to cooperate with the study, either initially or later on? We used questionnaires to probe indirectly some of their more conscious, verbally communicable motives both pro and con (Michaux, Michaux, Esser, and Oliver, 1968). We can supplement those findings with what we inferred from our personal acquaintance with subjects during data collection. Favorable (as well as unfavorable) attitudes to the hospital, enduring beyond discharge, appeared to generalize readily to the project. Underlying that process, and making for loyal cooperativeness, was an emotional dependence which typically embraced aftercare as well as the project and the hospital (Lipsitt, 1962; Scheflen, 1965). It contrasted strikingly with the separatism we have attributed to nonparticipants (Chapter II). In other subjects, a tendency akin to dependence was passive-submissiveness, often associated with perceiving the project in terms of authority and prestige (Jones, 1965). Again not far removed from these two tendencies was the need for help, coupled with perception of the evaluation relationship as helpful and, we believe, with the actual experience of benefit from participation (Rashkis, 1960).[4] Other motives for participating, though

[4]One important aspect of such benefit appeared to be a form of learning, verbally induced by repeated testing with the KAS. It is common clinical knowledge that many individuals, especially at lower levels of education and social class, are unable freely to recognize, describe, and discuss adjustment problems as such. The recurrent KAS sessions had the effect of providing such persons with verbal "handles" for taking hold of their experience at unfamiliar vantage-points. The process was not limited to patients, though informants naturally used it somewhat differently. Certain informants began to manifest discriminating awareness of patients' specific adjustment difficulties. They would then become more solicitously observant of the patients, thereby improving the informant-patient relationships and the patients' own chances for betterment. A few informants were so stimulated by the KAS and the stress inquiry that they even kept notes which they brought with them to their evaluation sessions. These phenomena

clearly discernible, seemed less central and/or less prevalent: altruism—helping us, helping other patients; narcissism—exhibitionism, pseudo-gregariousness; loneliness—the need to fill an empty life; and eroticism—occasionally directed quite openly at opposite-sex examiners.

The above remarks have dealt chiefly with patients, but informants were by no means always in the background. When the informant was the dominant member of the dyad, he often exerted decisive influence in the decision to participate or to refuse. The KAS and interview were approached quite seriously, but not necessarily completed more validly, by those informants who were intimately involved with patients—whether that involvement was one of concord or antagonism. Some informants turned in more favorable reports on patients (on the matching KAS scales) than did the same patients on themselves; in other cases the converse held true. Nurturing and cherishing attitudes toward patients were frequent among the former, bitterness and disparagement among the latter. Discrepancies in both directions are a fertile field for both treatment and research. We have admittedly slighted the topic in our data analysis.

reinforce our belief that the patient's close affiliate is a therapeutic resource whose potentials are often far from fully deployed. Furthermore, the KAS effects we have noted here suggest strongly that questionnaires of this kind could be strategically useful in programs of grass-roots mental health education. See Rashkis and Diggory (1963).

# References


American Psychiatric Association, Committee on Nomenclature and Statistics. 1952. *Diagnostic and statistical manual: mental disorders.* Washington, D.C.: American Psychiatric Association, Mental Hospital Service.

Angrist, Shirley; Dinitz, S.; Lefton, M.; and Pasamanick, B. 1961. Rehospitalization of female mental patients. *Arch. Gen. Psychiat.* 4: 363-70.

Barry, J. R., and Fulkerson, S. C. 1966. Chronicity and the prediction of duration and outcome of hospitalization from capacity measures. *Psychiat. Quart.* 40: 104-21.

Bonstedt, T., and Akdogu, U. F. 1961. Is symptomatic relief enough? *Hosp. Commun. Psychiat.* 17(1): 36-37.

Campbell, D. T. 1963. From description to experimentation: interpreting trends as quasi-experiments. In *Problems in Measuring Change*, ed. C. W. Harris, pp. 212-42. Madison, Wis.: University of Wisconsin Press.

Clausen, J. A. and Yarrow M. R., eds. 1955. *The impact of mental illness on the family.* Special edition of *J. Soc. Issues* 11: 3-65.

Dinitz, S.; Angrist, Shirley; Lefton, M.; and Pasamanick, B. 1961. The post-hospital psychological functioning of former mental hospital patients. *Ment. Hyg.* 45: 579-88.

Division of Occupational Analysis, U.S. Employment Service. 1949. *Dictionary of occupational titles: Volume II. Occupational classification and industry index.* 2d ed. Washington, D.C.: Government Printing Office.

Dohrenwend, B. P., and Dohrenwend, Barbara S. 1965. The problem of validity in field studies of psychological disorder. *J. Abnorm. Psychol.* 70: 52-69.

Edwards, A. L. 1960. *Experimental design in psychological research.* New York: Rinehart.

Engelhardt, D. M.; Freedman, N.; Glick, B. S.; Hankoff, L. D.; Mann, D.; and Margolis, R. 1960. Prevention of psychiatric hospitalization with use of psychopharmacological agents. *J. Amer. Med. Ass.* 173: 147-49.

Engelhardt, D. M.; Freedman, N.; Hankoff, L. D.; Mann, D.; and Margolis, R. 1963. Long-term drug-induced symptom modification in schizophrenic outpatients. *J. Nerv. Ment. Dis.* 137: 231-41.

Engelhardt, D.; Freedman, N.; and Mann, D. 1963. The influence of previous hospitalization on the clinical course of psychopharmacologically treated schizophrenic outpatients. *Comprehen. Psychiat.* 4: 337-42.

Freeman, H. E., and Simmons, O. G. 1963. *The mental patient comes home.* New York: Wiley.

Fuller, J. L. 1967. Experiential deprivation and later behavior. *Science* 158: 1645-52.

Gillis, L. S., and Keet, M. 1965. Factors underlying the retention in the community of chronic unhospitalized schizophrenics. *Brit. J. Psychiat.* 3: 1057-67.

Gordon, H. L.; Rosenberg, D.; and Morris, W. E. 1966. Leisure activities of schizophrenic patients after return to the community. *Ment. Hyg.* 50: 452-59.

Gorwitz, K. 1969. The demography of mental illness in Maryland. *Md. State Med. J.* 15: 40-49.

Gorwitz, K.; Bahn, Anita K.; Chandler, Caroline A.; and Martin, W. A. 1963. Planned uses of a statewide psychiatric register for aiding mental health in the community. *Amer. J. Orthopsychiat.* 33: 494-500.

Gorwitz, K.; Bahn, Anita K.; Klee, G.; and Solomon, M. 1966. Release and return rates for patients in state mental hospitals of Maryland. *Publ. Hlth Rep.*, 81: 1095-1108.

Greenblatt, M.; Levinson, D. J.; and Klerman, G. L., Eds. 1961. *Mental patients in transition: steps in hospital-community rehabilitation.* Springfield, Ill.: Charles C. Thomas.

Gross, M.; Hitchman, Irene L.; Reeves, W. P.; Lawrence, J.; and Newell, Pauline C. 1961. Discontinuation of treatment with ataractic drugs. In *Recent advances in biological psychiatry*, ed. J. Wortis, Vol. III, pp. 44-63. New York: Grune and Stratton.

Guy, W.; Hogarty, G.; and Gross, M. 1965. A model of research for emergent community mental health programs. *Amer. J. Orthopsychiat.* 35: 413-14. (Abstract)

Hankoff, L. D.; Engelhardt, D. M.; Freedman, N.; Mann, D.; and Margolis, R. 1960. Denial of illness in schizophrenic outpatients: effects of psychopharmacological treatment. *Arch. Gen. Psychiat.* 3: 657-64.

Harris, C. W., ed. 1963. *Problems in measuring change.* Madison, Wis.: University of Wisconsin Press.

Hogarty, G. E., 1966. Discharge readiness: the components of casework judgment. *Soc. Casewk.* 47: 165-71.

Hogarty, G. E., 1968. Hospital differences in the release of discharge ready chronic schizophrenics. *Arch. Gen. Psychiat.* 18: 367-72.

Hogarty, G. E.; Dennis, Helen; Guy, W.; and Gross, Gertrude M. 1968. "Who goes there?"—a critical evaluation of admissions to a psychiatric day hospital. *Amer. J. Psychiat.* 124: 934-44.

Hogarty, G. E.; Katz, M. M.; and Lowery, Henri A. 1967. Identifying candidates from a normal population for a community mental health program. In *Psychiatric epidemiology and mental health planning*, Monroe, R. D.; Klee, G. D.; and Brody, E. B., eds. Psychiatric Research Report 22, pp. 220-34. Washington, D.C.: American Psychiatric Association.

Hollingshead, A. B., and Redlich, F. C. 1958. *Social class and mental illness: a community study.* New York: Wiley.

Honigfeld, G., and Gillis, R. 1967. The role of institutionalization in the natural history of schizophrenia. *Dis. Nerv. Syst.* 28: 660-63.

Howard, K. I. 1964. Differentiation of individuals as a function of repeated testing. *Educ. Psychol. Measmt.* 24: 875-94.

Hughes, J. S., and Little, J. C. 1967. An appraisal of the continuing practice of prescribing tranquillizing drugs for long-stay psychiatric patients. *Brit. J. Psychiat.* 113: 867-73.

Hyman, H. 1955. *Survey design and analysis: principles, cases and procedures.* New York: Free Press.

Johnston, R., and McNeal, B. F. 1965. Residual psychopathology in released psychiatric patients and its relation to readmission. *J. Abnorm. Psychol.* 70: 337-42.

Jones, E. E. 1965. Conformity as a tactic of ingratiation. *Science* 149: 144-50.

Kandel, D. B., and Williams, R. H. 1964. *Psychiatric rehabilitation: some problems of research.* New York: Atherton Press.

Katz, M. M., and Lyerly, S. B. 1963. Methods for measuring adjustment and social behavior in the community: I. Rationale, description, discriminative validity and scale development. *Psychol. Rep.* 13: 503-35.

Katz, M. M.; Lowery, H. A.; and Cole, J. O. 1965. Behavior patterns of schizophrenics in the community. In *Explorations in typing psychotics*, ed. M. Lorr, pp. 209-31. Oxford: Pergamon Press.

Kintz, B. L.; Delprato, D. J.; Mettee, D. R.; Persons, C. E.; and Schappe, R. H. 1965. The experimenter effect. *Psychol. Bull.* 63: 223-32.

Kurland, A. A. 1954. Psychiatric research in a state psychiatric hospital. *Md. State Med. J.* 3: 611-14.

Kurland, A. A. 1962. The Spring Grove State Hospital research program. *Psychopharmacol. Serv. Ctr. Bull.* 2: 87-88.

Linder, F. E. 1966. The health of the American people. *Scient. American* 214 (6): 21-29.

Lipsitt, D. R. 1962. Dependency, depression, and hospitalization: toward an understanding of a "conspiracy." *Psychiat. Quart.* 36: 537-54.

Lorei, T. W. 1964. Prediction of length of stay out of the hospital for released psychiatric patients. *J. Consult. Psychol.* 28: 358-63.

Marks, J., Stauffacher, J. C., and Lyle, C. 1963. Predicting outcome in schizophrenia. *J. Abnorm. Soc. Psychol.* 66: 117-27.

Maryland Department of Mental Hygiene. 1966. *Annual statistical report for the fiscal year ending June 30, 1964.* Baltimore.

May, P. R. A.; Tuma, A. H.; and Kraude, W. 1965. Community follow-up of treatment of schizophrenia–issues and problems. *Amer. J. Orthopsychiat.* 35: 754-63.

McNemar, Q. 1962. *Psychological statistics.* 3rd ed. New York: Wiley.

Mechanick, P., and Nathan, R. J. 1965. Is psychiatric hospitalization obsolete? *J. Nerv. Ment. Dis.* 141: 378-83.

Michaux, Mary H.; Michaux, W. W.; Esser, Eugenie K.; and Oliver, Barbara A. 1968. Attitudes of psychiatric ex-patients toward a study of community adjustment. *Psychol. Rep.* 23: 567-72.

Michaux, Mary H.; Ota, Kay Y.; Hanlon, T. E.; and Kurland, A. A. 1963. Rater perseveration in measurement of patient change. *Educ. Psychol. Measmt.* 23: 171-84.

Michaux, W. W. 1959. Traumatic implications of psychiatric disability discharge from the armed services. *Milit. Med.* 124: 273-83.

Michaux, W. W.; Gansereit, Kathleen H.; McCabe, O. L.; and Kurland, A. A. 1967. The psychopathology and measurement of environmental stress. *Commun. Ment. Hlth. J.*, 3: 358-72.

Nickerson, K. S.; Epps. A. J.; and Heckel, R. V. 1966. Personal responsibility and psychoactive drug taking behavior in discharged mental patients. *Commun. Ment. Hlth. J.* 2: 202-4.

Orlinsky, Nancy, and D'Elia, E. 1964. Rehospitalization of the schizophrenic patient. *Arch. Gen. Psychiat.* 10: 47-54.

Pao, P. N. 1960. Young schizophrenic mothers' initial posthospital adjustment at home. *Arch. Gen. Psychiat.* 2: 512-20.

Park, L. C., and Lipman, R. S. 1964. A comparison of patient dosage deviation reports with pill counts. *Psychopharmacologia* 6: 299-302.

Peterson, D. B., and Olson, G. W. 1964. First admitted schizophrenics in drug era: follow-up Anoka schizophrenic cohort, 1956-1958. *Arch. Gen. Psychiat.* 11: 137-44.

Rahe, R. H.; McKean, J. D., Jr.; and Arthur, R. J. 1967. A longitudinal study of life-change and illness patterns. *J. Psychosom. Res.* 10: 355-66.

Rashkis, H. 1960. Cognitive restructuring: why research is therapy. *Arch. Gen. Psychiat.* 2: 612-21.

Rashkis, H. A., and Diggory, S. F. 1963. Perceptual organization and the development of insight. *Arch. Gen. Psychiat.* 9: 552-58.

Reilly, E. L.; Wilson, W. P.; and McClinton, Hortense K. 1967. Clinical characteristics and medication history of schizophrenics readmitted to the hospital. *Int. J. Neuropsychiat.* 3: 85-90.

Sargent, Helen D.; Modlin, H. C.; Faris, Mildred T.; and Voth, H. M. 1958. Situational variables. *Bull. Menninger Clin.* 22: 148-66.

Sargent, Helen D. 1960. Methodological problems of follow-up studies in psychotherapy research. *Amer. J. Orthopsychiat.* 30: 495-506.

Scheflen, A. E. 1965. The institutionalized, the institution-prone and the institution. *Psychiat. Quart.* 39: 203-19.

Schooler, Nina R.; Goldberg, S. C., Boothe, Helvi.; and Cole, J. O. 1967. One year after discharge: community adjustment of schizophrenic patients. *Amer. J. Psychiat.* 123: 986-95.

Shaffer, J. W.; Forbes, J. A.; and DeFelice, E. A. 1967. Some suggested approaches to the analysis of chronic toxicity and chronic drug administration data. *Toxicol. Appl. Pharmacol.* 10: 514-22.

Sherman, L. J.; Moseley, E. C.; Ging, Rosalie; and Bookbinder, L. J. 1964. Prognosis in schizophrenia: a follow-up study of 588 patients. *Arch. Gen. Psychiat.* 10: 123-30.

Smith Kline and French Laboratories. 1962. *A new chapter.* Philadelphia, Pa.

Summerfield, A., and Lubin, A. 1951. A square root method of selecting a minimum set of variables in multiple regression. *Psychometrika* 16: 271-84.

Tuerk, I., and Gorwitz, K. 1963(a). *Statistics newsletter No. IV-2.* Baltimore: Maryland State Department of Mental Hygiene.

Tuerk, I., and Gorwitz, K. 1963(b). *Statistics newsletter No. IV-4.* Baltimore: Maryland State Department of Mental Hygiene.

U.S. Department of Health, Education, and Welfare, and Maryland State Department of Mental Hygiene. 1964. *Maryland Psychiatric Case Register statistical series: annual tables for year ended June 30, 1963.* Bethesda, Md., and Baltimore.

U.S. Department of Health, Education and Welfare, and Maryland Department of Mental Hygiene. 1966. *Maryland Psychiatric Case Register Study of Patients Admitted to Three State Mental Hospitals 7/1/61 - 12/31/62.* Vols. 1 and 2. Baltimore.

Vaillant, G. E. 1964. Prospective prediction of schizophrenic readmission. *Arch. Gen. Psychiat.* 11: 509-18.

Williams, R. H. 1963. The strategy of sociomedical research. In *Handbook of medical sociology*, ed. H. E. Freeman. S. Levine, and L. G. Reeder, pp. 423-47. Englewood Cliffs, N.J.: Prentice-Hall.

Windle, C. 1954. Test-retest effect on personality questionnaires. *Educ. Psychol. Measmt.* 14: 617-33.

Windle, C. 1955. Further studies of test-retest effect on personality questionnaires. *Educ. Psychol. Measmt.* 15: 246-53.

Wing, J. K.; Monck, Elizabeth.; Brown, G. W.; and Carstairs, G. M. 1959. Morbidity in the community of schizophrenic patients discharged from London mental hospitals in 1959. *Brit. J. Psychiat.* 110: 10-21.

Yahraes, H. 1967. How do emotionally sick people get better? In *Mental health program reports*, ed. Office of Program Analysis, National Institute of Mental Health, Public Health Service Publication No. 1568, pp. 205-16. Bethesda, Md.: National Institute of Mental Health.

# Index

THE JOHNS HOPKINS PRESS

*Designed by Arlene J. Sheer*

*Composed in Press Roman text and display*
*by Jones Composition Company, Inc.*

*Printed on 55-lb. Perkins and Squier R*
*by Universal Lithographers, Inc.*

*Bound in Riverside Linen*
*by L. H. Jenkins Co., Inc.*